Pocket Guide to
Intravenous Therapy

Pocket Guide to Intravenous Therapy

Joanne C. LaRocca, R.N., M.N., C.D.E.

Clinical Nurse Specialist
St. Francis Regional Medical Center,
Wichita, Kansas

Shirley E. Otto, M.S.N., R.N., O.C.N.

Clinical Nurse Specialist
St. Francis Regional Medical Center,
Wichita, Kansas

with 50 illustrations

The C. V. Mosby Company

St. Louis • Baltimore • Toronto   1989

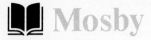
Mosby

Editor: Don Ladig
Assistant Editor: Audrey Rhoades
Production Editor: John Casey
Design: Rey Umali

Printed in the United States of America

The C.V. Mosby Company
11830 Westline Industrial Drive, St. Louis, Missouri 63146

Library of Congress Cataloging in Publication Data

LaRocca, Joanne C.
  Pocket guide to intravenous therapy.

  Bibliography: p.
  Includes index.
  1. Intravenous therapy. 2. Nursing. I. Otto,
Shirley E. II. Title. [DNLM: 1. Infusions, Intravenous—
handbooks. 2. Infusions, Intravenous—nurses' instruction.
WB 39 L326p]
RM170.L37 1989   615'.63   88-13256
ISBN 0-8016-5189-1
TSI/AG/AG   9 8 7 6 5 4 3

Nursing Consultants

Anne Marie Frey, B.S.N., C.R.N.I.
I.V. Nurse Clinician
St. Christopher's Hospital for Children
Philadelphia, Pennsylvania

Carolyn Hedrick, B.S.N., C.R.N.I.
Assistant I.V. Therapy Coordinator
Moses H. Cone Memorial Hospital
Greensboro, North Carolina

Mary J. Huizenga, R.N., B.A.G.E., M.A.Ed.
Nurse Educator
Blodgett Memorial Medical Center
Grand Rapids, Michigan

Sharon Kohler, R.N., B.S.N.
Coordinator, I.V. Therapy
Brigham and Women's Hospital
Boston, Massachusetts

Jane Scott, B.S.N.
Director of Nursing
Sac Osage Hospital
Osceola, Missouri

To staff nurses everywhere—especially those at St. Francis Regional Medical Center who have generously shared their hints along the way.

Preface

All health-care professionals are practicing in a rapidly changing, highly complicated environment in which IV therapy is a major treatment modality. Tremendous technological and reimbursement changes have necessitated proficiency in not only clinical skills but also documentation, patient teaching, and demonstration of quality assurance. Implantable ports, state-of-the-art pain management, and complex home IV medication regimens have challenged the nurse's practice climate. Increasingly, greater numbers of patients with serious illnesses, for example, AIDS, cancer, and end-stage organ diseases, require astute, long-term IV medication management. *Pocket Guide to Intravenous Therapy* has been designed to give nurses, working in diverse patient care settings and with varying clinical preparation, an easily accessible, accurate, and concise reference based on recognized national standards of practice.

The advent and increased use of multiple and diverse IV products and equipment in all settings have added a new dimension of complexity to the demands on the busy nurse. Now more than ever, advanced IV skills are sought by all nurses. For the nurse entering practice, returning to practice, or changing areas, learning these skills can be intimidating, and therefore a quick reference is needed. Home IV therapy, integration of nursing diagnoses into the care plan, and third party documentation demands may be a new or changing concept in some areas. This book features practical strategies and tools for patient teaching, sample documentation using nursing diagnoses, and nursing practice audits that can be readily adapted to all settings.

Each chapter discusses a major aspect of IV therapy. All chapters contain pertinent information, clinical alerts to clarify topics, tables for convenient reference, documentation recommendations, nursing diagnoses, patient/family teaching for self-management, home care considerations, and pediatric considerations. The content of the book has been organized in the manner in which nurses think and perform while providing care.

Chapter 1: Infusion Guidelines presents an overview of IV therapy principles.

Chapter 2: Venipuncture examines skills, product selection, and infection control issues.

Chapter 3: Central Venous Catheters contrasts and compares all the central venous catheters and provides step-by-step procedures for each device.

Chapter 4: Calculations for IV Therapy illustrates the use of all formulas required for accurate delivery of IV therapy.

Chapter 5: IV Fluids reviews the assessments and interventions required for the basic electrolytes. A table of replacement fluids is included.

Chapter 6: IV Medication Administration describes all modalities of IV medication administration. Information on the most frequently administered IV medications is included, as is a discussion of state-of-the art pain medication administration.

Chapter 7: Blood and Blood Component Administration discusses all components and transfusion reactions in readily available tables. Guidelines for home administration of blood products are included.

Chapter 8: Chemotherapy Administration explains theoretical information and nursing management for preparation, delivery, and disposal of cytotoxic drugs in the hospital or outpatient setting.

Chapter 9: Parenteral Nutrition explains assessment parameters and nursing intervention and emphasizes teaching needs for self-management.

Appendix: Nursing diagnoses frequently encountered with IV therapy are used with sample charting.

Bibliography: Each chapter has suggested readings for those desiring more information.

The authors are indebted to the following persons: our families for consistent encouragement and support; Dottie Ott for expert typing in every crunch; Ann Stern for providing a vision of professionalism and creating an atmosphere for it to flourish; coworkers at St. Francis Regional Medical Center for the many resources shared; representatives of the manufacturers of IV supplies and equipment for information and assistance; and Don Ladig and the editorial staff at The C.V. Mosby Company for guidance.

Joanne C. LaRocca
Shirley E. Otto

Contents

Infusion Guidelines

Intravenous (IV) therapy is used to treat a wide variety of patient conditions. Although 70% of hospitalized patients receive IV therapy daily, treatment extends beyond this population to outpatient settings, long-term care and home care for the infusion of medications and parenteral nutrition, and the infusion of blood and blood products. Therefore, as more illnesses are treated outside of acute care, nurses in all settings need to expand their IV therapy skills.

Despite basic similarities among various IV therapy settings, each situation calls for specialized skills. The more compromised patient or the more complex regimen requires more astute patient management.

This chapter focuses on observations required when administering IV infusions and on supplies and equipment commonly required for delivering IV infusion therapy.

Accurate Flow Rates

Achieving accurate flow rates is always an important concern in IV therapy because accuracy decreases the incidence of complications, for example, infiltration, phlebitis, loss of patency, and the metabolic and circulatory overload problems that can result from runaway infusions. Frequently a combination of factors causes fluctuations in flow rates. Time-taping fluid containers, using volumetric chambers or electronic pumps and controllers, and selecting the appropriate drop size all aid in establishing and maintaining accurate fluid delivery (Figure 1-1).

Observations

Nursing observations required to maintain an accurate flow rate include determining whether any mechanical factors interfere with

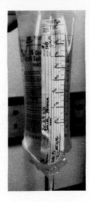

Figure 1-1
Infusion bag with time strip.
From Perry AG and Potter PA: Clinical nursing skills and techniques, St Louis, 1986, The CV Mosby Co.

fluid delivery, evaluating patient factors that can alter the flow rate, and observing for complications at the venipuncture site. The following mechanical factors may interfere with flow rate:

1. Positioning the fluid container less than 36 inches above the IV site does not allow gravity to overcome vascular pressure and thus prevents the infusion of IV fluids.
2. Kinks in either IV tubing or catheter tubing do not allow fluids to flow.
3. Taping at the catheter site can obstruct the catheter lumen particularly if a piece of tape is tightly placed directly over the bevel of the catheter.
4. Small-gauge catheters can slow fluid delivery and may require the use of a positive-pressure infusion device or replacement of the current IV catheter with one which has a larger gauge.

Patient factors such as the presence of tortuous veins and venous spasm can alter flow rates. Infiltration, phlebitis, and loss of patency may all occur at the IV site and terminate infusion.

Infusion System Evaluation

The following points should be considered during periodic evaluations of the entire infusion system:

1. IV is infusing at the prescribed rate.
2. All connections are intact.
3. The correct fluid is being infused.
4. IV tubing is placed correctly—not hooked on siderails or kinked.
5. Drop chamber contains the correct fluid level.
6. IV catheter is securely taped.
7. Tubing is checked and its replacement is considered.

Clinical Alert: Tubing needs to be changed according to the manufacturer's recommendations and in the following situations that reflect guidelines of the Centers for Disease Control and the Intravenous Nurses Society:

1. Routinely every 48 hours and when the IV catheter is changed
2. If the tip becomes contaminated from touch
3. If blood backs up in the tubing and is not immediately flushed out
4. Following piggyback administration of blood or lipid products

When the flow stops in tubing equipped with an in-line filter and no other cause can be found, the filter may need replacement.

Problems During IV Therapy

Most patients are able to assist with problems encountered during IV therapy if provided with the necessary information. Early identification of problems reduces the severity of most adverse outcomes. Listed below are troubleshooting tips and preventive measures for common IV problems.

Nursing Assessment	Nursing Intervention
Infiltration Infusion slows or stops Infusion device sounds occlusion alarm Tissue induration or swelling with cool tissue	Relocate IV site to other limb or above area of infiltration; if severe, apply warm compress *Prevention:* Observe site hourly during continuous infusions, especially if a positive-pressure pump is used

Continued.

Nursing Assessment	Nursing Intervention
Phlebitis Two or more of the following present: pain, redness, swelling, induration, cord	Relocate catheter to other limb or above area of phlebitis; if severe, apply warm compress *Prevention:* Filter solutions; rotate sites on a planned basis every 48 to 72 hours; secure catheter to prevent motion in vein
Runaway IV Dry IV or greater amount infused than scheduled	Notify physician and observe patient for signs of fluid overload and effects of IV additives *Prevention:* Recheck flow rate after changes; time-tape all infusions; use electronic pumps, controllers, or volumetric chambers for patients at greatest risk of developing complications
Sluggish IV Amount to be infused behind schedule	Observe entire system for mechanical or patient factors, for example, kinked tubing or patient lying on IV tubing; reposition or relocate IV device *Prevention:* Verify gauge of catheter is appropriate for type of infusion
Tubing disconnection Dampness from leaking fluid	Replace tubing if contamination occurs *Prevention:* Tape all connections or use locking devices for piggyback connections; use Luer-Lok connections for central venous catheters and other high risk situations, for example, patient is human immunodeficiency virus (HIV) seropositive
Blood backs up in tubing	Flush tubing with normal saline if blood backed up only briefly; change tubing if backup time is unknown *Prevention:* Place arm restraints below a venipuncture site; avoid dry IVs; keep fluid container 36 inches above site; teach patient not to raise arm above heart

Nursing Assessment	Nursing Intervention
IV line obstructed Resistance met when flushing attempted	Remove catheter or needle; do not force flush; relocate IV *Prevention:* Flush IV locks at least twice daily; in active children flush every 4 hours; change IV container before infusion running dry

Systemic Complications of IV Infusions

Although the majority of IV-related problems are localized to the infusion system or the catheter site, the following systemic complications can occur: circulatory overload, air embolism, foreign body embolism, and septicemia.

Circulatory overload

Symptoms: Dyspnea, cough, pitting edema in dependent areas, puffy eyelids, weight increase during the past 24 hours

Treatment: Decrease IV rate, elevate the patient's head, dangle feet if possible, check vital signs frequently, assess breath sounds for presence of moist crackles, contact the physician

Complications: Congestive heart failure and pulmonary edema

Possible cause: The patient has a history of compromised cardiac or renal condition, liver disease, or cerebral damage; an IV solution was inadvertently infused at a rapid rate; or the patient has received saline solution in excessive amounts, especially at night when renal function is normally reduced

Air embolism

Symptoms: Chest pain, shoulder pain, shortness of breath, cyanosis, low back pain, hypotension, weak pulse, loss of consciousness

Treatment: Immediately place the patient on left side in Trendelenburg position and contact the physician; stay with the patient, take vital signs, and consider oxygen administration; keep the IV site open

Complications: Shock and death

Possible cause: Inadvertent entry of air into the venous system, a greater problem with central lines than peripheral IVs; use Luer-Lok connections for all central lines

Foreign-body embolism

Symptoms: Same as for air embolism; this is a rare complication

Treatment: Immediately place the patient on left side in Trendelenburg position and contact the physician; take vital signs; apply tourniquet to extremity above the venipuncture site to confine embolus to the effected extremity; stay with the patient

Complications: Occlusion of blood flow to a body part; shock and death

Possible cause: Portion of the IV catheter was severed or another foreign body such as hair or a needle fragment inadvertently entered the IV catheter

Septicemia

Symptoms: Sudden or gradual rise in temperature, chills and shaking; increased pulse and respiratory rate, headache, nausea and vomiting, diarrhea

Treatment: Symptomatic as ordered by the physician; NOTE: Save IV catheter, tubing, and solution for possible culture; if IV supply is suspect, follow steps for alerting manufacturer of need for a product recall; establish another IV site for administration of drugs

Complications: Septic shock and death

Causes: Contamination of IV product(s), break in aseptic technique, especially in immunocompromised patients

Common Infusion-Related Supplies and Equipment

Supplies and equipment commonly required for IV therapy include IV poles, labels for the infusion container and IV tubing, tape, armboards, administration sets, filters, and flow regulation devices. Each IV admixture needs a label listing the following information: patient's name and identification number; additives, strengths, and amounts; primary solution and total volume; flow rate; preparation and expiration dates; storage requirements (when applicable), and identification of the person preparing and hanging the infusion. Each tubing should also be labeled with information on the date and time hung and the initials of the person hanging the tubing.

Selecting an Administration Set

Because many options are available in IV tubings, the IV set chosen depends on the needs of the particular situation. Some important considerations are mentioned below.

Drop size

Drop chambers deliver either microdrops (60 drops/ml) or macro-
drops (10 to 15 drops/ml). A macrodrop system should be selected
when large quantities of solution or fast rates are required.

Vents

Vents permit air to enter the vacuum in the bottle and to displace
the solution as it flows out. Unlike rigid glass containers, flexible
IV containers do not require vents. The tubing that is appropriate
for either the flexible or rigid IV container should be selected.

IV ports

Ports are required to administer secondary infusions and medications. Continuous-flow sets are designed with a back-check valve
that allows a piggyback to run and the solution to begin infusing
again after the piggyback is completed.

Volumetric chamber

Volumetric chamber IV sets are used to deliver small doses of
medication or fluid over an extended period of time. They are used
frequently with children and in intensive care settings to reduce the
risk of large amounts of fluids infusing too rapidly.

IV Filter Considerations

Infusion-related phlebitis is a common occurrence and may result
from particulates and microbes in the IV system or irritation caused
by the IV catheter. IV filters are designed to remove particulates
and microbes from IV infusions. However, filters are designed to
complement IV therapy and not replace aseptic technique.

Filtering may be done in a pharmacy area before delivery to the
patient care area or with a filter attached to the IV tubing. Filter
sizes range from 5 μm to 0.22 μm. The 0.45 μm filter may have an
air-eliminating capacity, but like the 0.5 μm to 5 μm filters, it

retains particulate matter. However, the 0.22 μm filter removes all particulate matter, fungi, and bacteria and is also air eliminating. The benefits of in-line filters and add-on filters have not been universally supported. However, no studies have contraindicated filter use, and many strongly encourage it. Problems associated with filters include clogging that may slow or stop the flow rate when debris accumulates on the filter surface; drug binding to the surface of the filter that may occur with some drugs, for example, insulin and amphotericin B; and adding unnecessary cost to basic IV systems when filters may not be indicated for short-term infusions.

Flow Control Devices

Flow rates can be regulated with clamps, accessory devices, and IV pumps and controllers.

Clamps

Every IV administration set has one or more clamps to regulate flow. Roller clamps adjust tubing diameter and restrict or increase the flow rate. A slide clamp either stops or starts IV flow and should not be used in conjunction with a roller clamp.

Accessory devices

Small-accessory flow-regulation devices may be added to administration sets to control the drop rate more precisely than a roller clamp. Most of these devices depress a larger area of tubing than do roller clamps, although they are less precise than electronic pumps and controllers.

IV pumps and controllers

Electronic devices deliver fluids with the highest degree of accuracy. Their ability to sound an alarm when an occlusion occurs may assist with early identification of flow problems. A pump has the ability to add pressure to an infusion under conditions of restricted flow. Controllers do not add pressure to the line to overcome resistance. (Pumps and controllers are discussed more completely in Chapter 6.)

Infection Control Practices

Patient Protection

Patients may be exposed to IV-related infections in a variety of ways. Nosocomial infections are best prevented when nurses wash their hands before making contact with any part of IV systems. Product and equipment contamination may occur during manufacture, storage, or therapy. If there is a break in aseptic technique during the course of therapy, tubing should be changed immediately, since the patient is at risk of developing a systemic infection. Potential sources of patient infection are summarized below.

Source of Contamination	Protective Measures
Manufacture or storage	Verify integrity of all packaging before use; discard a cracked bottle; check IV solutions against a light and a dark background for particulate matter; check expiration dates on packaging
Break in aseptic technique during therapy	Avoid touch contamination when spiking bags, priming tubing, or adding medications; change tubings if touch contamination occurs; disconnected equipment should not be reconnected
Blood in tubing	Flush IV immediately when blood backs up or change tubing if the time since backed up unknown; teach patients not to raise arm with IV above heart; do not use IV for routine blood drawing

Nurse Protection from IV-Related Infection

Traditionally, protection from IV-related infections has been considered only in relation to the patient. Concerns of nurses and other health-care workers of acquiring the HIV virus led the Centers for

Disease Control to develop guidelines for persons who perform invasive procedures. According to these guidelines, gloves should be worn when working with IV infusions, since there is a potential for contact with the patient's blood; hands should be washed before and after working with IV systems and immediately if hands are accidentally soiled with blood; and nurses need to be evaluated for exposure to infection if a needle stick or a blood splash occurs.

Documentation Recommendations

Records

Records are maintained to provide an accurate and easily retrievable account of patient care and treatment. Complete records are a principal means of communication among health-care team members. Increasingly, records are used by insurers to justify supply and equipment costs, by review organizations to evaluate quality of care, and by courts for malpractice claims. Therefore IV therapy

				I.V. SITE								
						SHIFT CHECK						
DATE	TIME	I.V. NO.	TUBING # CHANGE	INSERTION SITE	7--3	3—11	11—7	INFUSION DEVICE	VOLUME-SOLUTION-ADDITIVE-REMARKS	D/C	RATE	INITIALS

Signature	Initials	Signature	Initials	Signature	Initials

must be accurately and completely documented. Efficient chart forms can facilitate complete, concise documentation. IV therapy easily lends itself to flow sheet documentation.

Documentation Elements of Infusion Therapy

- Date and time of tubing changes; list all accessory tubings
- Date, time, and contents of IV fluids
- IV flow rate, including subsequent rate changes
- Electronic equipment used to regulate the flow
- Regular site assessments
- Presence of any complications and action taken to correct the problem
- Time IV therapy was discontinued, and whether the catheter was intact when removed
- All patient teaching and a reflection of understanding of instructions through return demonstration or repeating information

Labeling IV Containers

In addition to documentation in the patient record, specific information needs to be placed on labels attached to the IV container. All IV containers should be labeled with the patient's name and identification number, the name of the IV solution, a list of additives (including dosage), the date and time hung, initials of the person hanging the infusion, and the expiration date or time of the infusion.

Nursing Diagnoses

- Infection, potential for, related to invasive procedure
- Injury, potential for, related to obstruction of catheter
- Skin integrity, impaired: actual
- Fluid volume excess: actual or potential
- Fluid volume deficit: actual or potential

Patient/Family Teaching for Self-Management

Patients need to know the purpose of their therapy, the approximate duration of the treatment, and any movement restrictions that should be observed during the course of the infusion. In addition, patients should be taught to recognize and report the early signs and symptoms of infiltration or phlebitis. When electronic infusion devices are used, the patient should be instructed to call the nurse when an alarm sounds. Teaching activities to encourage patient cooperation and participation in care include the following measures:

- Discuss the signs and symptoms of possible infiltration or phlebitis, for example, swelling, pain, burning, soreness, redness, or a cool feeling at the insertion site.
- Teach the importance of reporting symptoms to the nurse.
- Discuss the importance of not readjusting the flow rate or bending or lying on the tubing.
- Show the patient how to avoid placing pressure on the venipuncture site when attempting to sit up in bed, pushing the IV pole, and positioning the arm with the IV catheter.
- Demonstrate how to wash the arm and hand in the area of the IV to ensure that the IV remains clean and dry.

Home Care Considerations

Before an electrolyte infusion is initiated in the home setting the patient must be in a stable condition and recent (past 24-hour) serum electrolyte values are recommended.

Patients and family or other caregivers who will manage infusions at home require extensive information related to management of all IV supplies and equipment. Storage requirements, infusion preparation, disposal of supplies, and management of all electronic equipment must be thoroughly understood before self-management is attempted. Return demonstrations and written instructions are needed for all aspects of care that the patient or family will be managing. Emergency phone numbers are crucial. In addition, patients and families need information on unusual findings that need to be reported, for example, adverse effects, phlebitis, and infiltration.

Pediatric Considerations

A child's total body water is greater than an adult's in proportion to size and is located mainly in the extracellular space. Therefore fluid and electrolyte balance in children differs from that in adults. Because a child has more body surface in proportion to body mass, greater fluid losses may occur, making dehydration the most common fluid imbalance in children.

The younger the child is, the more rapidly fluid and electrolyte imbalances develop. Therefore the following precautions are important:

- All pediatric infusions should be regulated with volumetric chambers or electronic devices to ensure accurate fluid delivery.
- Intake and output records should be maintained during IV therapy.
- The IV site and all equipment should be checked at least hourly.
- When restraints are required, make plans to hold the child frequently; allow the child as much freedom of movement as possible, and involve the parents in the child's care.

Chapter

Resources

What is IV therapy?

This information has been compiled to answer patients' commonly asked questions about IV therapy. It explains the IV procedure, why IV therapy is used, what a patient feels while receiving IV therapy, and precautions patients should observe to make their IV therapy go smoothly.

IV stands for *intravenous,* meaning inside the vein. For IV therapy, a catheter (a soft plastic tube about the size of a needle) or needle is inserted into a vein, usually in your hand or arm. The catheter or needle is attached to tubing and a fluid container that provide a way to give you medications and fluids.

How long will the IV stay in?

Your IV therapy may last only a few hours or up to several days. Your physician decides the duration of IV therapy.

Is IV therapy painful?

When the IV infusion is initiated, you will feel the insertion of the needle placing the catheter into your vein. As the IV solution enters your vein, it may sting for a few minutes, but the discomfort should stop in a short time.

If you feel any discomfort after the initial insertion, ask your nurse to check your IV site. Once the IV system is in place and secured, it should cause you minimal, if any, discomfort.

Is it possible to walk around?

If you have permission to get out of bed, you may do so even while receiving IV therapy. If your IV is being regulated by a pump

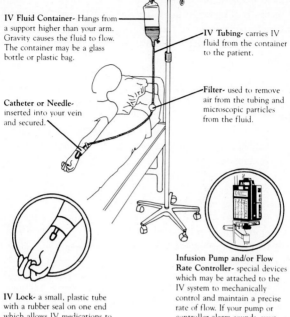

IV Fluid Container- Hangs from a support higher than your arm. Gravity causes the fluid to flow. The container may be a glass bottle or plastic bag.

IV Tubing- carries IV fluid from the container to the patient.

Catheter or Needle- inserted into your vein and secured.

Filter- used to remove air from the tubing and microscopic particles from the fluid.

IV Lock- a small, plastic tube with a rubber seal on one end which allows IV medications to be given intermittently.

Infusion Pump and/or Flow Rate Controller- special devices which may be attached to the IV system to mechanically control and maintain a precise rate of flow. If your pump or controller alarm sounds, your nurse will attend to the device.

or controller, ask your nurse to unplug the instrument before getting up. It will be plugged in again when you return to bed.

While you are up and walking, the pole should be pushed slowly with your free arm while holding your arm with the catheter lower than the level of your heart. Keeping your IV arm lower than your heart prevents blood from backing up into the tubing and keeps the IV flowing at the correct rate. Never take the IV bag off the pole.

Is bathing or showering allowed?

Depending on the type and location of your IV therapy, you may be allowed to shower or take a tub bath. Check with your nurse for permission or instructions regarding bathing or showering.

What is intermittent IV therapy?

When continuous IV fluids are not needed, your IV catheter is disconnected from the IV tubing, and an IV lock is attached to it. The IV lock is a device that allows IV medications to be given as needed.

What could the patient do to help?

Observing the following precautions will help your IV procedure go smoothly:

- Promptly report problems such as unusual swelling, redness, tenderness, or burning at the catheter site to your nurse.
- Do not touch any of the clamps or controls on the IV tubing. Ask the nurse to make all adjustments.
- Do not remove the fluid container from the IV pole.
- Be careful not to pull on the IV tubing.
- Minimize your arm movements, particularly at the joints closest to the catheter site.
- Do not raise your arm too high; the catheter site must be below the IV fluid container for it to flow properly.
- Do not lie on your arm or any part of your body receiving the IV.
- Avoid lying on the tubing or letting it get tangled in the bed.
- Ask for help. Many tasks can be difficult with an IV. Your nurse will be glad to assist you.

What happens after the IV is removed?

Immediately after your IV catheter is removed, pressure will be applied to the spot to seal the vein. After that, you may use your arm as you normally would.

If you have further questions about your IV therapy ask your nurse or physician.

Infusion Therapy Audit

	Yes	No	NA
The collection of data about the health status of a patient will be recorded and retrievable.			

Record Review

1. All IV solutions are sequentially recorded on the Infusion Record.
2. IV rates including rate changes are documented on the Infusion Record.
3. IV controller or pump use is documented at least every 24 hours according to agency policy.
4. Each shift documents a venipuncture site assessment on the Infusion Record.
5. Flushes are documented in conjunction with IV medication administration.
6. IV tubing changes are documented at least every 48 hours on the Infusion Record.

Patient Observation

1. IV solution hanging corresponds to the physician's order, information on Infusion Record and patient care plan.
2. IV has a time strip marked in hourly increments. NOTE: Includes IVs regulated by controllers or pumps
3. Time strip is initialed by the nurse hanging the bag.
4. The solution is being infused on time, within 30 minutes of schedule.
5. IV tubing is labeled with time of last tubing change.

Continued.

Infusion Therapy Audit—cont'd

	Yes	No	NA
The Patient's Educational Needs Will Be Addressed			
1. Patient has been instructed not to adjust flow rate of IV. "Did the nurses tell you not to make any adjustments to your IV?"			
2. Getting out of bed: "What have you been told about getting out of bed with your IV?"			
3. Controller/pump: "What have you been told to do if the alarm sounds?"			
4. Patient has been informed to report complications of IV therapy to the nurse. "What have you been told to report to your nurse?"			

Venipuncture

Venipuncture is a skill that is basic to IV therapy and can be learned and developed through frequent practice. Thorough understanding of both vein location and the venipuncture procedure increases confidence. Important elements of the procedure include patient preparation, vein selection, device selection, accurate insertion technique, knowledge of troubleshooting, and patient instruction.

Patient Preparation

Checking the patient's record for allergies and reviewing the physician's order and available laboratory results should be completed before approaching the patient. Supplies should be selected according to the purpose and duration of therapy and the patient's age and physical condition.

Patients who are unfamiliar with IV therapy may be frightened. When the patient is tense, the veins can constrict and make the venipuncture more painful and more difficult. Extreme anxiety can be lessened by instructing the patient to inhale and exhale slowly, to avoid looking at the IV site, and to focus on a pleasant image. These steps encourage patient cooperation:

1. Assume a confident attitude.
2. Greet the patient by name.
3. Introduce yourself.
4. Validate the patient's identification.
5. Explain the procedure in a way easily understood by the patient.
6. Ask for the patient's cooperation in holding his hand as still as possible.

Vein Selection

As a general rule, distal veins of the hands and arms should be used initially and subsequent venipunctures should be proximal to previous sites. Veins commonly used for IV therapy include the basilic, cephalic, and metacarpal (Figure 2-1). The extremity should be observed and palpated before a vein is chosen. Resiliency and location should be checked, and the vessel should be verified as a vein and not an artery. The differences between veins and arteries include the following qualities:

Veins	Arteries
Dark-red blood	Bright-red blood
Slow blood return	Rapid, pulsating blood return
Valves at point of branching	No valves
Flow toward heart	Flow away from heart
Superficial location	Deep location surrounded by muscle
Multiple veins supply an area	Single artery supplies an area

Observe the following guidelines for vein selection:
1. Use distal veins first.
2. Use the patient's nondominant arm if possible.
3. Choose a vein above areas of flexion.
4. Select a vein that is large enough to allow adequate blood flow around the catheter.
5. Always choose soft, full, unobstructed veins when available.

The following types of veins should be avoided if possible:
1. Previously used veins
2. Veins injured by infiltration or phlebitis
3. Sclerotic veins
4. Veins of a surgically compromised limb, for example, following a mastectomy or placement of a dialysis access
5. Areas of flexion, including the antecubital fossa
6. Leg veins, since circulation is sluggish and complications are more frequent
7. Small, thin-walled branches of main arm veins

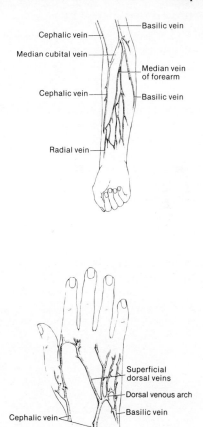

Figure 2-1

Venous anatomy.

From Perry AG and Potter PA: Clinical nursing skills and techniques, St Louis, 1986, The CV Mosby Co.

Venipuncture Device Selection

Choosing the correct device is as important to the outcome of the therapy as choosing the best vein. Improved product design has resulted in flexible, over-the-needle catheters that are appropriate for most applications of IV therapy (Figure 2-2). A dual-lumen peripheral catheter requires only one venipuncture and therefore is useful when the patient needs two different infusions (Figure 2-3). The separate lumens may be used to deliver potentially incompatible fluids such as intermittent antibiotics and an aminophlylline infusion.

Considerations when choosing a catheter include the size and condition of the vein selected, the viscosity of the fluid to be infused, the patient's age, and the expected length of therapy.

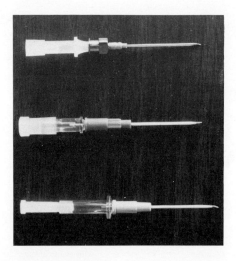

Figure 2-2
Over-the-needle cannulae.
Courtesy Alton Ochsner Medical Foundation, New Orleans.

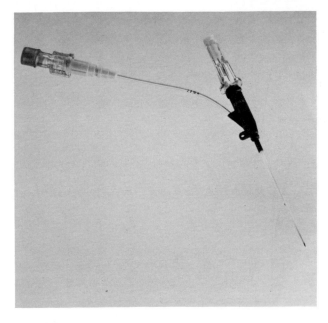

Figure 2-3
Arrow dual-lumen catheter.
Courtesy Arrow International, Inc, Reading, Pa.

Consult the following list when selecting a catheter gauge:
1. 16 gauge—major surgery or trauma
2. 18 gauge—blood and blood products, administration of viscous medications
3. 20 gauge—most patient applications
4. 22 gauge—most patient applications, especially children and the elderly
5. 24 gauge—pediatric patients and neonates

Clinical Alert: Choose the shortest catheter with the smallest gauge appropriate for the type and duration of the infusion. The larger the gauge number, the smaller the bore of the catheter.

Insertion Technique

Vein Location

To locate a suitable vein, apply a tourniquet 4 to 6 inches above the proposed site. The tourniquet should be tight enough to stop venous blood flow but not arterial flow. To encourage vein distention, ask the patient to clench and unclench his fist several times. When venous fill is difficult to achieve, placing the arm in a dependent position or applying warm packs may help alleviate the problem. The vein should then be stabilized, since stabilization of the vein before sticking is a key to successful venipuncture.

If the patient has a great amount of hair on his arm, clip the hair before venipuncture rather than shaving it, since shaving may nick the skin and create a potential site for infection.

Catheter Insertion

1. Clean the skin from the center outward with an approved solution (povidone-iodine, tincture of iodine, or 70% alcohol) and allow to dry (Figure 2-4).

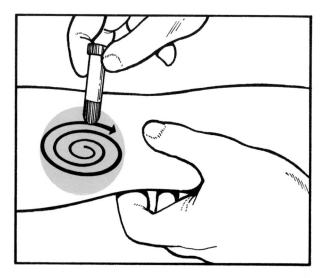

Figure 2-4
Cleansing the venipuncture site. Gloves should be worn during this procedure.

2. Apply a flat, soft tourniquet 4 to 6 inches above the site.
3. Anchor the vein; place your thumb over the vein to prevent movement and to stretch the skin taut against the direction of insertion.
4. Puncture the vein; hold the flash chamber of the catheter, not the hub; *A. direct approach*—place the needle bevel up at a 30- to 45-degree angle from the patient's skin (Figure 2-5); insert in the direction of venous flow; enter the vein; you may feel a "pop" and see a blood flashback; *B. indirect method*—enter the skin beside the vein and then direct the catheter to enter the side of the vein until you see a blood flashback.
5. Lower the needle until almost flush with the skin.

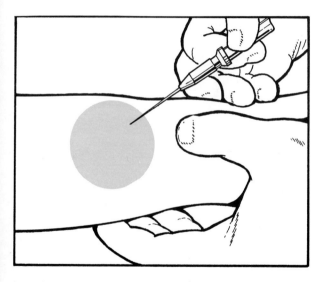

Figure 2-5

Catheter insertion. Insert catheter bevel side up at 30- to 45-degree angle in direction of blood flow. Gloves should be worn during this procedure.

6. Advance the catheter into the vein an additional ¼ to ½ inch before removing the stylet; release skin tension, hold the stylet, and advance the catheter (Figure 2-6).
7. Release the tourniquet and remove the stylet.
8. Apply primed tubing or an intermittent injection cap.
9. Tape the IV catheter and tubing into place (Figure 2-7).
10. Apply a sterile dressing.
11. Label the site (Figure 2-8).

Clinical Alert: When a stick is unsuccessful, use a new catheter for a second attempt.

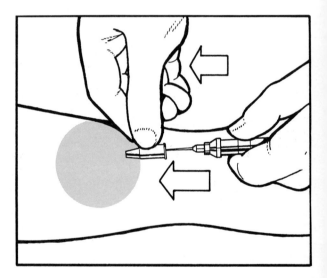

Figure 2-6
Advance catheter until blood flashback is seen. Gloves should be worn during this procedure.

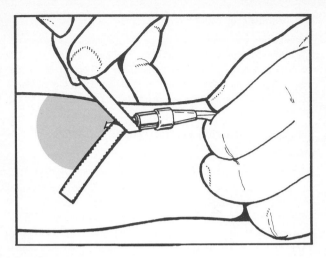

Figure 2-7
Anchoring the catheter. Gloves should be worn during this procedure.

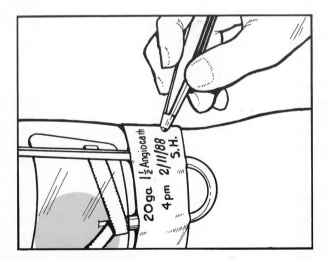

Figure 2-8
Label insertion site with catheter gauge, date and time of insertion, and initials of person performing the procedure. Gloves should be worn during this procedure.

Site Rotation

Venipuncture sites need to be changed on a planned basis every 48 to 72 hours to reduce the potential of phlebitis and infiltration. If the device remains in place longer than 72 hours because of limited vein selection, the reason should be documented in the patient's record. A new site is chosen by moving up the patient's arm, or in a proximal direction.

Peripherally Inserted Central Venous Catheters
Catheter description

Peripherally inserted central venous catheters are available for insertion by nurses with advanced IV therapy skills as an alternative to physician-placed central venous catheters. These Silastic catheters may vary in length, gauge, and number of lumens. Selection depends on the intended use, for example, duration of venous access and administration of vesicant chemotherapeutic agents and parenteral nutrition.

Catheter insertion

Insertion of peripheral central venous catheters is performed with strict aseptic technique by nurses who have been validated in the procedure. Usually the catheters are inserted peripherally via the basilic or the cephalic vein. Before a multilumen catheter insertion, each lumen must be heparinized before introduction into the vein. The distal lumen of the catheter containing a siliconized wire stylet to assist in catheter advancement does not require heparinization. An introducer may be used for ease of insertion and threading of the catheter into the vein. The catheter should be advanced slowly into the vein to avoid destruction of the vein intima. Following placement, the catheter is secured with sutures and covered with a sterile dressing. Placement is verified by a radiograph before infusion of medications or fluids.

Catheter maintenance

Refer to *Chapter 3—Central Venous Catheters*—for catheter maintenance procedures.

Venipuncture for Laboratory Sampling

Blood samples are most commonly drawn from an antecubital vein using vacuum collection devices. The antecubital is selected because the veins are large and have thicker walls than the veins that are lower in the arm and hand. When antecubital veins are not available, samples are drawn using a butterfly needle attached to a syringe, since the vacuum containers collapse the smaller veins. **Clinical Alert:** Draw blood samples from the arm without an IV whenever possible, since laboratory values may be altered by the IV fluids. If laboratory samples are drawn from the arm with an IV, stop the infusion for 1 to 2 minutes before drawing the blood sample.

Tips for Difficult Veins

When difficult veins are encountered, it should be remembered that systematic preparation is the key to a successful stick. The patient should be in a comfortable position with his arm lowered (or use hot towels to help distend his veins). A confident attitude should be assumed while the patient is reassured. Slapping the vein is rarely helpful because it makes the skin red, causes irritation over the vein, and makes the patient more tense.

Interventions to increase successful sticks in difficult situations are listed below.

Nursing Assessment	Nursing Intervention
Obese patient; unable to palpate or see veins	Create a visual image of the venous anatomy; select a longer catheter
Fragile skin and veins, infiltration occurs after stick	Use minimal tourniquet pressure; if bounding pulse, do not use tourniquet
Vein rolls when stick attempted	Anchor vein with thumb while sticking
Patient is in shock or has minimal venous return	Leave tourniquet on to promote venous distention; use 16- or 18-gauge catheter

Infection Control Concerns

Patient Considerations

Infection at the venipuncture site is usually caused by a break in aseptic technique during the procedure. The following measures reduce patient risk:

1. Wash hands before starting an IV or working with the IV equipment.
2. Use an approved antiseptic to clean the patient's skin.
3. Clip hairs at the venipuncture site.
4. Do not reuse a catheter or needle.
5. Apply a sterile dressing to the site.

If an infection is found at a venipuncture site, for example, purulent drainage or cellulitis, the following care is required:

1. Culture the drainage before removing the catheter.
2. Remove the catheter by holding the hub so the portion of the catheter under the skin is not touched.
3. Hold the catheter over a sterile container and use sterile scissors to cut the distal portion of the catheter so that it falls into a sterile container (Figure 2-9).
4. Label the container and send it to the laboratory.
5. Restart the IV using all new supplies—including the tubing and solution.

Nurse Considerations

Both HIV and hepatitis virus are blood borne. When performing the venipuncture procedure, it is important for the nurse to adhere to the Centers for Disease Control guidelines for invasive procedures. Recommended practices for nurses involved with IV therapy include the following:

1. Consider IV needles as potentially infective. Do not recap needles after use. Have a puncture-resistant container at the bedside for disposal of used needles.
2. Wear gloves when inserting IV needles or handling tubings.
3. Wash hands thoroughly and immediately if they are accidentally contaminated with blood.

If a needle stick or a blood splash occurs, the nurse needs to be evaluated as soon as possible after exposure and periodically thereafter. Each professional needs to be acquainted with new information related to epidemiology, modes of transmission, and prevention of HIV and other blood-borne diseases. Further, the nurse should incorporate into daily practice universal precautions concerning blood, body fluid, and secretions.

Documentation Recommendations

The following information is recorded on the patient's dressing:
- Nurse's initials
- Date and time of procedure
- Catheter or needle gauge

The following information is documented in the patient's record according to agency policy:
- Date and time of venipuncture

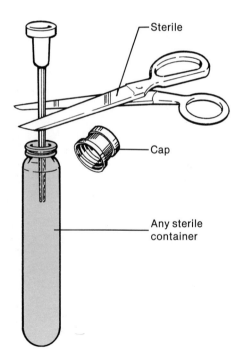

Figure 2-9
Culturing an IV catheter.

- Number of attempts required
- Site location
- Catheter gauge and length
- All IV supplies used
- IV fluids and flow rate, if infusion initiated
- Presence of any complications and actions taken to correct the problem
- Patient teaching and a reflection of understanding

ndx Nursing Diagnoses

- Skin integrity, impaired: potential related to catheter insertion
- Infection, potential for, related to break in skin, contamination of supplies, or break in sterile technique at time of venipuncture
- Anxiety related to invasive procedure
- Comfort, altered: pain, associated with procedure or complications at insertion site

Patient/Family Teaching for Self-Management

Patients who are receiving IV therapy need to receive information that will enable them to protect their IV site and to report complications to the nurse. Information should include the following:

1. Movement restrictions
2. Information to be reported
   a. Redness, swelling, or discomfort at site
   b. Blood in tubing
   c. Moisture on the dressing
   d. IV not infusing or infusion device alarms
3. Changing of the IV site (every 48 to 72 hours or immediately if complications occur)
4. How to bathe with the IV site

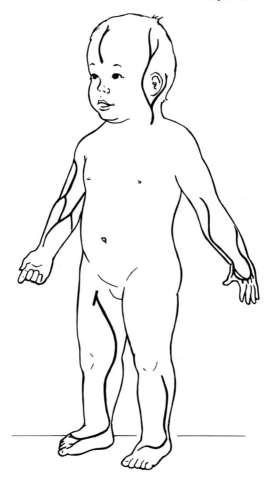

Figure 2-10
Superficial veins used most often for IV infusion in infants and very young children.
From Kempe CH, Silver HK, O'Brien D, and Fulginiti VA, editors: Current pediatric diagnosis and treatment, ed 9, Los Altos, Calif, 1987, Appleton & Lange.

Home Care Considerations

- Demonstrate catheter removal to the patient and caregiver in case it becomes accidentally dislodged.
- Instruct the patient in the frequency and technique of flushing the intermittent injection lock.
- Teach the patient to recognize signs of phlebitis and infiltration: presence of redness, induration, swelling, or pain. Inform the patient of the planned frequency of IV site rotation.

Pediatric Considerations

- The dorsal surfaces of hands and feet are the most frequently selected sites (Figure 2-10).
- The dorsal vein of the hand allows the child the greatest mobility.
- Always select a site that will require the least restraint.
- Scalp veins are very fragile and require protection so that they are not infiltrated easily—used for neonates and infants.

Chapter
Resources

Quality Assurance Monitoring—Universal Blood and Body Fluid Precautions to Minimize AIDS Transmission

	Yes	No	NA
1. Gloves are worn for touching blood and body fluids, mucous membrane, or non-intact skin of all patients.			
2. Gloves are worn for handling items or surfaces soiled with blood or body fluids.			
3. Gloves are worn when staff member has a break in her skin.			
4. Gloves are *not worn* when 1, 2, or 3 above is not present or likely, for example, transporting patients.			
5. Gloves are worn for performing venipuncture and other vascular access procedures.			
6. Hands are washed immediately after gloves are removed.			
7. Hands or other skin surfaces are washed immediately and thoroughly if contaminated with blood or other body fluids.			
8. Used sharps, such as needles or scalpels, are placed in biohazard needle box.			
9. Needles are *not* purposely bent, broken, or recapped.			
10. Needle container is not overfilled.			
11. Disposable wastes and articles contaminated with blood or large amounts of body fluids are placed in impervious containers for a trash pickup.			
12. Spills of blood or body fluids are cleaned up with a 1:10 solution (prepared daily) of Clorox and water.			

Continued.

Quality Assurance Monitoring—Universal Blood and Body Fluid
Precautions to Minimize AIDS Transmission—cont'd

	Yes	No	NA
When the nurse is exposed to procedures that are likely to generate splashes or droplets, the following precautions should be implemented.			
1. Masks and protective eye wear are worn during procedures that are likely to generate droplets of blood or body fluid, for example, nasotracheal suctioning, to prevent exposure of mucous membrane.			
2. Gowns are worn during procedures that are likely to generate splashes of blood or other body fluids, for example, wound irrigation, patient bowel or bladder incontinence.			
3. Reusable items, for example, suction bottles and oxygen setups are emptied with care to avoid splashing.			
4. All soiled linen is placed in laundry bag. Bag is *not* overfilled.			
5. Patients with diarrhea—there is no change in practice by staff member whether a patient has been diagnosed as having AIDS or not.			
6. Patients who are coughing—there is no change in practice by staff member whether a patient has been diagnosed as having AIDS or not.			

Venipuncture Audit

	Yes	No	NA
1. Verify physician order.			
2. Check appropriate laboratory data.			
3. Check allergy data.			
4. Calculate flow rate.			
5. Choose and set up appropriate equipment: solution, set, venipuncture device.			
6. Wash hands.			
7. Correctly label IV with patient name, IV additives, rate of administration.			
8. Introduce self to patient.			
9. Assess patient identification.			
10. Explain procedure to patient and answer patient questions appropriately.			
11. Choose appropriate vein: location, size, condition.			
12. Apply tourniquet without occluding arterial flow.			
13. Cleanse area according to agency policy.			
14. Perform venipuncture according to accepted procedure using no more than two attempts.			
15. Attach tubing to IV cannula and establish flow of solution.			
16. Anchor needle and apply dressing to venipuncture site according to accepted procedure.			
17. Label venipuncture site with date, catheter gauge, catheter length, and nurse's initials.			
18. Set flow rate according to prescribed rate.			
19. Check for infiltration.			
20. Place IV pole on same side of bed as IV site.			
21. Record procedure in patient record according to agency policy.			

Central Venous Catheters

3

Long-term venous access without repeated venipunctures is required for persons with a variety of medical conditions, including cancer, chronic bowel disease, and long-term antibiotic therapy. The critically ill patient is a potential candidate for a central venous catheter, since the catheter provides access to essential IV therapy. Central venous catheters are commonly used to administer all types of IV therapy, including chemotherapy, hyperalimentation, antimicrobial agents, and blood component therapy. These catheters may also be used for blood sampling. Indications for inserting the catheters continue to increase because research has shown low complication rates with well-maintained catheters.

The versatility of the catheters allows the patient to receive treatment in a variety of health-care settings. In any such setting the nurse is a key member of the team responsible for delivering fluids and drugs to patients. Whatever the purpose of insertion, safe and proper care from the nurse ensures successful use and catheter longevity. (See Table 3-1 for types and characteristics of central venous catheters.)

Insertion

Catheter insertion is usually performed by a physician with the patient under local anesthesia. Sterile technique is maintained during the procedure. The catheter is inserted via percutaneous placement or a venous cutdown procedure. It is then threaded into the subclavian or jugular vein or the superior vena cava at its junction with the right atrium. A subcutaneous tunneling procedure or suturing of the catheter is used to secure catheter placement. Before administration of IV fluids or drugs, a catheter-imaging radiograph is recommended to confirm catheter placement.

Text continued on p. 42.

Table 3-1   Central venous catheters

Types of Catheters	Characteristics
Subclavian catheter single and multilumen (dual-, triple-, quadruple-lumen available)	Short-term use (less than 60 days) Polyurethane and Silastic material Sutured in place Volume 0.5 to 0.6 ml/lumen Sterile dressing required for duration of catheter placement Allows simultaneous administration of potentially incompatible medication and fluids (applies to the multilumen catheter *only*) Requires heparinization of each lumen every 12 hours Can be repaired if damaged

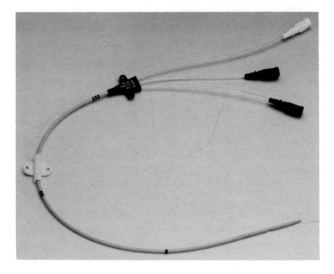

Multilumen subclavian catheter.
Courtesy Arrow International, Inc, Reading, Pa.

Continued.

Table 3-1 Central venous catheters—cont'd

Types of Catheters	Characteristics
Right atrial catheters single-, dual-, triple-lumen, for example, Hickman-Broviac catheters	Long-term use (1 to 2 years) Silastic material Subcutaneously tunneled in place Dacron cuff Volume 1.8 ml/lumen uncut adult catheter Sterile environment until exit site healed; after exit site healed, dressing optional Requires scheduled flushings with heparinized saline when not in use Repair kits available

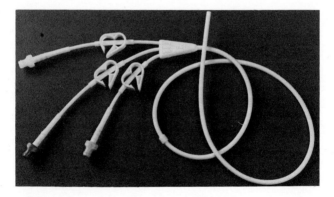

Hickman® catheter.
Courtesy CR Bard, Inc, Cranston, RI.

Central venous catheter with three-position valve and closed distal tip, for example, Groshong catheter	Same as right atrial catheter except it requires scheduled flushings with normal saline when not in use NOTE: Always *vigorously* flush the Groshong catheter. Do *not* clamp catheter following flushing. Repair kits available

Table 3-1   Central venous catheters—cont'd

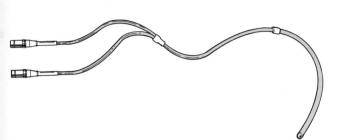

Groshong central venous catheter.
Courtesy Catheter Technology Corp, Salt Lake City, Utah.

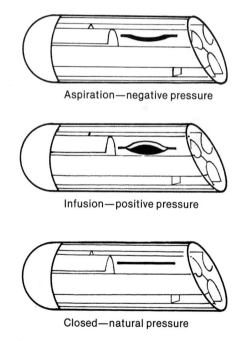

Aspiration—negative pressure

Infusion—positive pressure

Closed—natural pressure

Three-position Groshong valve.
Courtesy Catheter Technology Corp, Salt Lake City, Utah.

Continued.

Table 3-1   Central venous catheters—cont'd

Types of Catheters	Characteristics
Implantable ports venous placement single- and dual-lumen	Long-term use (1 to 2 years) Metal or plastic portal chamber with silicone septum connected to Silastic catheter Self-sealing silicone septum allows up to 2000 punctures Portal chamber sutured and catheter tunneled in place Requires Huber needle in place for port access

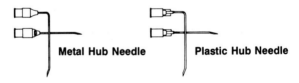

Cross section of implantable port with needle access.
Courtesy Pharmacia Deltec, Inc, St Paul, Minn.

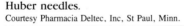

Metal Hub Needle   **Plastic Hub Needle**

Huber needles.
Courtesy Pharmacia Deltec, Inc, St Paul, Minn.

Clinical Alert: The implantable port is also available for epidural, intraarterial, and intraperitoneal placement. Administer IV fluids only through the *venous* port. Use other sites only for infusions of medications of fluids specific to that placement site. Be sure to check the product information accompanying each port for instructions and use (Figure 3-1).

Table 3-1   Central venous catheters—cont'd

Types of Catheters	Characteristics
Implantable ports	Volume 2 ml port and lumen (adult)
	Maintain sterile environment when port accessed
	Port requires at least monthly heparinization
	Minimal self-care requirements
	Nurse and patient instructional material available from manufacturers
	Does not require a dressing when not in use.

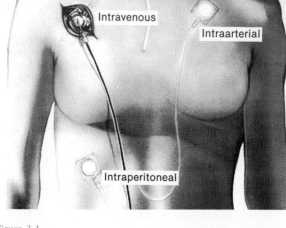

Figure 3-1
Placement of IV, intraarterial, and intraperitoneal port.
Courtesy Pharmacia Deltec, Inc, St Paul, Minn.

Critical Elements of Nursing Management of Central Venous Catheters

Aseptic Technique

Strict aseptic technique is required to maintain venous integrity and to prevent serious infection. A rubber-topped Luer-Lok cap is used to provide a sterile closed system when the catheter is not directly connected to IV tubing. This cap must fit securely to prevent any contamination or loss of blood. All tubing, needle junctions, or injection caps must be prepared with povidone-iodine before needle insertion to prevent introduction of microorganisms into the catheter.

Infection Control

Nurse protection regarding infection control recommendations includes disposing of needles or blood contaminated caps and tubings into puncture-resistant containers; wearing gloves during catheter management procedures, for example, blood sampling; and washing hands thoroughly and immediately if accidentally contaminated with blood.

Catheter Maintenance Procedures

Catheter maintenance procedures may vary from one setting to another and according to each manufacturer's recommendations. The specific protocol for each device should be consulted before use. The following suggestions are within the guidelines of each product's requirements:

  I. Site care
    A. Change gauze dressing every 24 hours.
    B. Change bioocclusive dressing every 3 to 5 days or more frequently to maintain an occlusive seal.
    C. Coil right atrial catheter and tape securely to skin when catheter is not in use.
  II. Cap change (depends on the frequency of catheter access)
    A. Change subclavian catheter every 3 to 7 days.
    B. Change right atrial catheter every 7 days.
    C. Change cap when rubber coring occurs.
    D. Change cap at dressing change or catheter flushing.

III. Needle and tubing change for implantable port
   A. Change sterile needle and tubing for each bolus access.
   B. Change sterile needle and tubing for continuous infusion every 5 to 7 days.
IV. Blood sampling
   A. To ensure a pure blood sample from multilumen catheters, turn off IV fluids 1 full minute before blood or fluid discard.
   B. Recommended discard for laboratory samples should equal three times the volume of each catheter lumen (range 2 to 6 ml) for all the central venous catheters.
   C. Obtain laboratory sample.
   D. Flush catheter immediately with normal saline or heparin solution.
   E. Resume previous catheter function or heparin lock the device.
V. Heparinization—The volume and concentration of the heparin solution and frequency of flushing remain a controversial issue in catheter patency management.
   A. Volume
      1. Between 1 and 2 ml per catheter/lumen (child) for right atrial catheter and implantable port
      2. Approximately 2.5 ml per catheter/lumen (adult) for right atrial and subclavian catheters
      3. Approximately 5 ml for implantable port (adult)
   C. Concentration—heparin (10 to 1000 units/ml)
   D. Frequency
      1. Subclavian catheters: every 12 to 24 hours
      2. Right atrial catheters: daily to weekly
      3. Implantable ports: monthly
   E. To ensure a heparin lock, maintain a positive pressure (keep a forward motion on the syringe plunger as needle is removed from cap or port) while injecting the heparin solution into the catheter to prevent a back-flow of blood into the catheter tip.

Accessing an Implantable Port

Since the port is located beneath the skin surface, the boundaries specific to each device and the resilience of the silicone septum need to be known before needle access. This procedure requires aseptic technique using sterile supplies.

1. Wash hands and apply gloves.
2. Cleanse portal site with povidone-iodine swabs, starting over the portal and moving outward in a spiral motion to cover an area 5 inches in diameter.
3. Attach tubing with Huber needle to syringe filled with saline.
4. Locate the portal septum by palpation (Figure 3-2).
5. Insert the needle perpendicular to the septum and push it slowly but firmly through the skin and portal septum until it comes to rest at the bottom of the portal chamber.
6. Aspirate for a blood return; flush the system with normal saline to confirm that fluid flows through the system.
   a. Note any unusual resistance to flow or any swelling around the injection site, since either may be a sign of insufficient needle penetration, incorrect needle placement, catheter blockage, or a leaking portal system, catheter, or connection.
   b. For bolus injection of medication, remove the empty saline syringe, replace it with the drug-filled syringe, and administer the injection. At the completion of the injection, flush the catheter with normal saline and then heparin lock the device while withdrawing the needle from the portal septum (Figure 3-3).
   c. For a continuous infusion, remove the empty saline syringe, replace with IV infusion tubing, and secure tubing. Since the Huber needle remains in the portal chamber

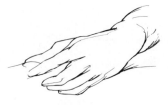

Figure 3-2
Palpating the implantable port.
Courtesy Pharmacia Deltec, Inc, St Paul, Minn.

during the infusion, secure the needle to prevent inadvertent dislodgment by placing a 2 × 2 gauze dressing underneath the needle and applying antibacterial ointment around the needle site. Finally, apply a semipermeable occlusive dressing over the entire area. Secure extension tubing to minimize needle dislodgment (Figure 3-4).

Clinical Alert: Use Huber needle at a 90-degree bend for continuous infusion.

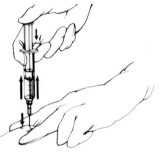

Figure 3-3
Bolus injection into implantable port.
Courtesy Pharmacia Deltec, Inc, St Paul, Minn.

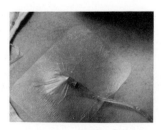

Figure 3-4
Continuous infusion with implantable port.
From Perry AG and Potter PA: Clinical nursing skills and techniques, St Louis, 1986, The CV Mosby Co.

Table 3-2   Troubleshooting tips—central venous catheters

Nursing Assessment	Nursing Interventions
Deeply implanted port	Note portal chamber scar
Unable to palpate port	Use deep palpation technique or seek assistance of second person to locate port
Do not feel needle stop against portal chamber	Use 1½- or 2-inch Huber needle
Unable to obtain blood return	Try to change catheter alignment by raising the patient's arm on same side as catheter
	Roll the patient to opposite side
	Ask the patient to cough, sit up, take a deep breath
	Try infusing 10 ml of normal saline into catheter
	Reaccess catheter or implantable port with new sterile needle
Unable to inject fluid or medication	Follow above steps (''Unable to obtain blood return'')
	If unable to inject fluid or obtain blood return, notify the physician
	Catheter placement should be determined by radiographic examination

Table 3-3   Potential complications—central venous catheters

Nursing Assessments	Nursing Interventions
Air embolus	Clamp central line
May occur during connections or disconnections of syringes and IV tubing	Instruct the patient to lie on left side with head down; Trendelenburg position
	Notify the physician

Table 3-3   Potential complications—central venous catheters—
cont'd

Nursing Assessments	Nursing Interventions

Air embolus
  Symptoms
    Chest pain
    Cyanosis
    Increased pulse and respirations
    Decreased blood pressure
	Monitor vital signs
	Remain with the patient
	Administer O_2
	Initiate peripheral IV

Catheter dislodgment Medication or fluid leaking from catheter or exit site	Note presence or absence of suture in securing subclavian catheter or Dacron cuff protruding from exit site of right atrial catheter Report finding to physician Secure catheter and extension tubing with tape
Catheter migration Unable to inject fluid or medication	Notify physician to determine catheter placement
Catheter occlusion Unable to inject fluid or medication	Gently flush catheter with appropriate normal saline flush *Do not use force* (Catheter may rupture) Notify the physician; there is a potential need for injection of fibrinolytic agent Inject urokinase 1 ml (5000 units/ml) into catheter port using a tuberculin syringe After 10 minutes, try to aspirate the clot If necessary, repeat aspiration at 5-minute intervals for 30 minutes Upon establishing catheter patency, withdraw 5 ml of fluid and discard before flushing catheter lumen

Continued.

Table 3-3   Potential complications—central venous catheters—cont'd

Nursing Assessments	Nursing Interventions
Catheter occlusion	with normal saline; resume previous catheter function or heparin lock the device
	Declotting procedure may be repeated using two doses of the fibrinolytic agent; wait 1 hour between procedures
Catheter sepsis	Culture catheter exit site, port site, and extension tubing, and obtain a blood sample from peripheral site
Inflamed, reddened, painful catheter exit or port site	
Purulent exudate	Notify physician
Elevated temperature	Administer appropriate prescribed antibiotics
	Do not access an inflamed port site
Vessel thrombosis	Notify the physician to determine catheter placement via radiograph
May be related to diameter of catheter in relation to patient's vessel size	
Symptoms	
Edema and tenderness of neck, shoulder, and arm on the same side as the catheter	

Documentation Recommendations

- Daily assessment of port or exit site, skin or catheter integrity, and catheter placement
- Procedure access for each catheter or device
- Heparinization or normal saline flush—drug, dose, volume, date, and time
- Injection cap or extension tubing changes
- Site care management
- Patency of catheter, blood sampling, and infusion of medications or fluids

- Patient symptoms related to catheter malfunction or potential complications associated with central venous catheter
- Patient/family education regarding understanding (verbalized or return demonstration) of catheter self-care management

Nursing Diagnoses

- Skin integrity, impaired: potential related to erosion of skin at exit site or frequent implantable port access
- Injury, potential for, related to venous obstruction, catheter dislodgment, catheter migration, or catheter occlusion
- Infection, potential for, related to contamination of supplies, break in sterile technique when managing catheter, performing site care, accessing catheter, or dressing changes
- Knowledge deficit regarding ongoing self-management of catheter

Patient/Family Teaching for Self-Management

- Assess the patient's ability and willingness to learn, availability of caregiver, home environment, and previous experience or expectations.
- Describe purpose and function of the catheter or device.
- Instruct the patient regarding preoperative and postoperative procedures.
- Explain self-care management issues: site care, changing injection cap, and flushing catheter with heparin solution or normal saline require demonstration to facilitate learning and integration of necessary skills.
- Review symptoms related to each potential complication with emergency self-management techniques and reporting of that information immediately to the physician.
- Reinforce the troubleshooting tips related to potential catheter malfunctions with appropriate intervention strategies.
- Provide information on obtaining, storing, and disposing of supplies and availability of 24-hour hotline for problems.

Home Care Considerations

- Keep supplies and equipment used for catheter management in a secure place.

- Schedule daily or intermittent catheter flushings at the same time every day to coincide with the patient's activities of daily living.
- Reinforce to the patient or caregiver to report abnormal findings immediately to the physician, such as elevated temperature, inflamed port or exit site, catheter malfunction, and unusual discomfort related to catheter.
- Discard all supplies used for catheter care into a puncture resistant container, for example, an empty coffee can, in preparation for garbage pick up.

Pediatric Considerations

Right atrial catheters and implantable ports are used in children for administration of antibiotics, chemotherapy, total parenteral nutrition, and blood sampling. The heparin concentration, volume of flush for each lumen, and flushing frequency of the catheters need to be correlated with the child's body surface area (BSA) requirements. Teaching self-care management strategies should include consideration of the child's growth and development status.

Chapter
Resources

MULTILUMEN SUBCLAVIAN CATHETER CARE
Patient Information

This catheter is composed of pliable polyurethane material and allows easy access to your vascular system (bloodstream). Because of its unique design (three separate ports), more than one medication or IV fluid can be given at one time. The catheter is used for short-term situations (usually 2 to 8 weeks) to give medication or for blood sampling. It is inserted by a physician using sterile technique, under a local anesthetic. Catheter placement is usually checked by getting a radiograph at the end of the procedure. The catheter is held in place by sutures securing the small wing-tip device next to the skin. It is important to keep this area free of germs.

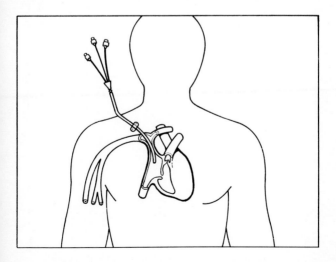

Site care

The exit site area must be cleansed on a daily basis with a cleansing agent such as povidone-iodine (Betadine) or alcohol. Be careful to clean around the sutures and remove any old drainage (see illustration below). The exit site is covered with a transparent or a

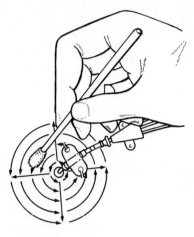

sterile gauze dressing (4 × 4) to keep the catheter in place. Tape the dressing securely (see illustration below).

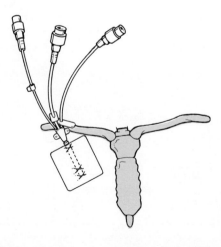

Catheter heparinization—flushing the catheter

Flush each catheter port every 12 or 24 hours with heparinized saline (Tubex) 2.5 ml (100 units/ml).

- Gather supplies: Povidone-iodine/alcohol swabs
  Heparin Tubex 2.5 ml (100 units/ml)
  Heparin Tubex syringe
- Wash hands with soap and water for 10 seconds.
- Prepare heparin Tubex syringe.
- Cleanse catheter cap with povidone-iodine followed by alcohol swab.
- Insert heparin Tubex syringe into catheter port; push with a forward motion on the syringe plunger to inject the heparin into the catheter.
- Continue pressing on the plunger as you withdraw the needle.
- Discard used heparin Tubex.

(Patient and/or family member needs to demonstrate with return demonstration the use of heparin Tubex syringe.)

Catheter cap

The catheter caps must be changed on a weekly basis or if cap is contaminated or cored. The nurse will assist you with this on your visits to the office.

Reminders

- Call the physician if you have signs of infection or fever: redness, swelling, tenderness, or drainage around the catheter.
- If your catheter resists the solution, do not force the solution into the catheter; change position, and if resistance continues, stop and call your physician.
- Keep sharp objects away from the catheter; if the catheter is accidently cut or punctured, clamp tightly by folding the catheter back on itself and securing with a rubber band or a clamp; immediately call your physician to report the problem.

GROSHONG CATHETER

Patient Information

This catheter is composed of a transparent silicone rubber and allows easy access to your vascular system (bloodstream). Because its unique design (a patented two-way slit valve next to a rounded, closed tip), it requires minimal catheter care. The catheter may have a single- double- or triple-port and is usually in place months to two years. It is inserted by a physician using sterile technique, under a local anesthetic. Catheter placement is usually checked by getting a radiograph at the end of the procedure. A Dacron fiber cuff is placed below the skin to hold the catheter in place and to prevent infection.

Site care

The area around the exit site of the catheter must be kept *sterile* and covered with a dressing for the first seven days after insertion. Thereafter the exit site needs to be cleaned on a daily basis with povidone-iodine swabs or alcohol wipes.

Sterile procedure

During the first seven days of catheter insertion, wash hands thoroughly with soap and water. Remove old dressing and discard. Apply sterile gloves. Cleanse the exit site with sterile povidone-iodine swabs or alcohol wipes. Be careful to clean around the

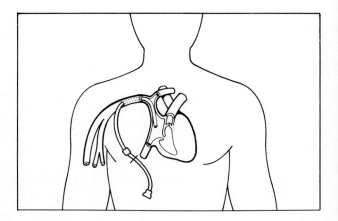

sutures and remove any old drainage. The exit site is then covered with a transparent or sterile gauze dressing (4 × 4) to keep the catheter in place.

Daily procedure (use when catheter exit site has healed)

Wash hands thoroughly. Cleanse exit site with povidone-iodine swabs or alcohol wipes. Cleanse catheter with alcohol wipe from exit site to injection cap. Tape catheter in place.

Flushing the catheter

Flush the catheter every seven days with 5 ml of normal saline. Wash hands with soap and water for 10 seconds. Prepare 5 ml normal saline syringe. Cleanse catheter with povidone-iodine swabs followed by alcohol wipes. Insert needle into Luer-Lok injection cap. Continue pressing in the syringe plunger as you withdraw the needle. Discard needle and syringe into (coffee can) container.

Catheter cap

The cap must be changed every seven days. Wash hands with soap and water for 10 seconds. Unscrew old cap. Replace with new cap and secure tightly.

Reminders

- Call your physician if you have signs of infection or fever: redness, swelling, tenderness, or drainage around the catheter.
- If there is resistance in flushing the catheter, alter your position (lean forward, breathe deeply, cough), and then continue flushing catheter.
- If unable to inject normal saline into the catheter, call your physician promptly.

HICKMAN CATHETER

Patient Information

The Hickman catheter is a flexible silicone tube that gives easy access to your vascular system (bloodstream). The catheter can be used to draw blood for laboratory samples or to give chemotherapeutic drugs and other medications, IV fluids, blood or blood components, and nutritional suppport. The catheter is inserted under local anesthesia—you cannot feel it inside your body. With the aid of a radiograph fluoroscope, the catheter is placed into your upper chest and directed to the upper right chamber (right atrium) of your heart. After insertion, the catheter is sutured into place. A Dacron fiber cuff is placed below the skin to hold the catheter in place and to prevent infection. When you no longer need the catheter, it can be removed by your physician or nurse.

Catheter care

Taking care of your catheter is a simple but serious process. If you follow the preparation steps carefully, you can avoid complications and problems.

Your main responsibility is to help keep the catheter clean. When the catheter is not being used for drawing blood samples or giving medication, it is filled with a medication called heparin. This solution cleanses the catheter and keeps blood from clotting in it.

You must flush your catheter with heparin as directed by your physician. Each time you receive medications or have blood drawn, your catheter must be flushed.

Always keep your hands and work area clean when working with the catheter. Always use a brand new needle and syringe. Cleanliness prevents infection.

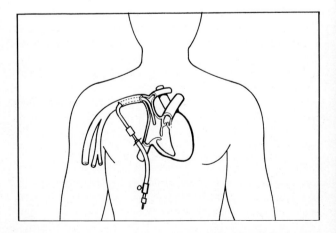

Daily catheter care

- Clean the area around the catheter with an alcohol wipe and check the area for redness or swelling.
- Release catheter clamp, if clamp is in place.
- Clean the rubber cap on the catheter with a povidone-iodine wipe.
- Insert the syringe needle into the rubber cap.
- Inject the solution slowly; if you feel any resistance, change your position by raising your arm, leaning forward, or taking a deep breath; if resistance continues, remove the needle and call your physician.
- Remove the needle after injecting the solution and discard both the needle and the syringe; these should be used only once.
- Coil the catheter and tape securely to skin. Do not let the catheter hang loosely.

Supplies

Your physician or nurse will give you a list of supplies needed to care for your catheter. The supplies are available at your pharmacy and may include:

- Povidone-iodine or alcohol wipes
- Syringes and needles
- Heparin solution
- Dressing supplies

Reminders

- If your catheter resists the solution, do not force the solution into the catheter. First, check for clamped catheter, and then, alter your position (lean forward, cough, or breathe deeply). If resistance continues, stop and call your physician.
- Each day, inspect the skin around the catheter for redness, swelling, tenderness, or drainage. These signs, along with fever, may indicate infection. If any of these signs occur, call your physician promptly.
- Keep scissors and sharp objects away from the catheter. If the catheter is accidentally cut or punctured, tie it in a knot or clamp it between the puncture site and your chest and call your physician immediately.
- After the incision has healed (approximately 2 weeks), you may participate in your regular activities as long as the catheter is taped securely to your chest.

Calculations for IV Therapy

4

Flow Rate Calculations

Flow rate calculations are integral to the safe delivery of IV fluids and medications. Information necessary to calculate the flow rate includes the following:

1. Volume of fluid to be infused
2. Total infusion time
3. Calibration of the administration set used (number of drops per milliliter it delivers; this information is found on the IV tubing package)

Manufacturers of IV tubings use 10, 12, 15, 20, or 60 drops (gtt) to deliver a milliliter (ml) of fluid. To calculate an *hourly* IV rate, use the following formula:

$$\frac{\text{gtt/ml of set}}{60 \text{ min}} \times \text{total hourly volume} = \text{gtts/min}$$

1000 ml over 8 hours = 125 ml/hr; 10 gtt/ml infusion set   Equation 1

$$\frac{10\text{gtt/ml}}{60 \text{ min}} \times 125 \text{ ml/hr} =$$

$$\frac{10 \text{ gtt}}{60 \text{ min}} = \frac{1}{6} \div \frac{125 \text{ ml/hr}}{1} = \frac{1}{6} \div \frac{125}{1} = 20 \text{ gtt/min}$$

Since $^{10}\!/_{60}$ reduces to $^1\!/_6$, any hourly volume may be divided by 6 to determine the drops per minute of an IV set that delivers 10 drops per milliliter.

1000 ml over 10 hours = 100 ml/hr; 15 gtt/ml infusion set   Equation 2

$$\frac{15 \text{ gtt/ml}}{60 \text{ min}} \times 100 \text{ ml/hr} =$$

$$\frac{15 \text{ gtt}}{60 \text{ min}} = \frac{1}{4} \div \frac{100 \text{ ml/hr}}{1} = \frac{1}{4} \div \frac{100}{1} = 25 \text{ gtt/min}$$

Clinical Alert: Calculations for other IV tubing sets include: gtt/ml/infusion set

$$\frac{12 \text{ gtt}}{60 \text{ min}} = \text{⅕ or divide by 5}$$ Equation 3

$$\frac{15 \text{ gtt}}{60 \text{ min}} = \text{¼ or divide by 4}$$

$$\frac{20 \text{ gtt}}{60 \text{ min}} = \text{⅓ or divide by 3}$$

$$\frac{60 \text{ gtt}}{60 \text{ min}} = 1 \text{ or divide by 1}$$

Often a 24-hour volume is prescribed by a physician. Divide the desired volume by 24 before using the above formula.

3000 ml/24 hr   Equation 4

3000 ÷ 24

$$\frac{3000}{1} \times \frac{1}{24} = 125 \text{ ml/hr}$$

To calculate drops per minute for fluid volume that is prescribed milliliters per hour, proceed to the step of

$$\frac{\text{gtt/ml of set}}{60 \text{ min}} = \text{total hourly volume} = \text{gtt/min}$$ Equation 5

When small-volume IV piggyback medications are administered through the same IV line as a continuous infusion, the IV infusion will *not* stay on time unless the *time* needed to infuse the piggyback medications is included in the total calculations. Substract the time required for the piggyback infusion from the 24-hour period before calculating the drops per minute for the continuous IV.

IV fluid 3000 ml 24 hr   Equation 6

Piggy back medication

50 ml over 20 min × 3 in 24 hr = 1 hour

24 hr − 1 hr = 23 hrs

3000 ml ÷ 23

$$\frac{3000}{1} \times \frac{1}{23} = 130 \text{ ml/hr}$$

This consideration is important for very ill patients receiving triple antibiotic therapy, especially if each drug dose is diluted in 50 to 100 ml of IV fluid.

Monitoring IV flow rate is facilitated by recording the milliliter per hour by hourly increments on each IV container. This information may be recorded on the IV time-tape affixed to the outside of the container.

Flow Rate	Time
.0 ml	8 AM start
125	9
250	10
375	11
500	12 PM
625	1
750	2
875	3
1000 ml	4 PM end

Subsequent rate adjustments can be made throughout the IV fluid delivery by observing the desired milliliters to be infused at the scheduled time and adjusting the flow rate.

Drug Dose Calculations—Adult

IV drug dosage may be prescribed in microgram/kilogram/minute (μg/kg/min), milligram/hour, units of drug per hour, or by body surface area (BSA) requirements. Calculations of μg/kg/min include conversion of pounds to kilograms and milligrams to micrograms. Drug units per hour and milligrams per hour are determined by the concentration of a drug in a volume of solution. BSA requirements are calculated via a nomogram. The following formulas and examples describe a step-by-step process for each method.

Microgram/Kilogram/Minute

Convert weight in pounds to kilograms (divide the weight by 2.2):

132 lb ÷ 2.2 = 60 kg

Convert total milligram medication dose to microgram (multiply the milligram by 1000 or move decimal three places to the right)

100 mg × 1000 = 100,000 μg

In most instances a microdrop IV tubing will be used, and 60 microdrops per minute equal 1 milliliter.

Patient—176 lb Equation 7

Medication—Dopamine 200 mg in 250 ml dilute strength (DS)/0.45 normal saline

Dose—Dopamine 5 μg/kg/min

1. Convert 176 lb to kg

$$176 \div 2.2 = 80 \text{ kg}$$

Dopamine 200 mg to micrograms

$$200 \text{ mg} \times 1000 = 200,000 \text{ μg}$$

2. Determine μg/minute dose base on kg weight

$$5 \text{ μg/kg/min} \times 80 \text{ kg} = 400 \text{ μg/min}$$

3. Determine μg/ml dosage

$$200,000 \text{ μg}:250 \text{ ml} = x \text{ μg}:1 \text{ ml}$$

$$\frac{200,000}{250} = \frac{x}{1}$$

$$x = \frac{200,000}{250}$$

$$x = 800 \text{ μg/ml}$$

4. Determine microdrops per minute

   microdrop tubing 60 mgtt/ml

   800 μg: 60 microdrops = 400 μg/min

$$\frac{800}{60} = \frac{400}{x} :: 800 \text{ x} = 24,000$$

$$x = \frac{24,000}{800}$$

$$x = 30 \text{ microdrops/min}$$

Milligram/Hour

Drug concentration milligrams per milliliter will vary according to the dilution factor. Note the concentration milligrams per milliliter of each drug before calculation of flow rate.

Morphine—50 mg in 1000 ml = 1 mg/20 ml   Equation 8

Dose—Morphine 4 mg/hr

Infusion set—60 gtt/min

1 mg = 20 ml

4 mg = x ml/hr

$4 \times 20 = 80$

80 ml/hr

$\dfrac{60 \text{ microdrops}}{60 \text{ minutes}} \times 80 \text{ ml/hr} = \text{microdrops/min}$

$\dfrac{60}{60} \times 80$

$1 \times 80 =$

80 microdrops/min

Units of Drug per Hour

Heparin—20,000 units in 500 ml dextrose in water (D/W) Equation 9

Dose—heparin 1000 units/hr

Infusion set—60 gtt/ml

20,000 units heparin ÷ 500 ml infusion

$20,000 \div 500 = x$ units/ml

$x = \dfrac{20,000}{500}$

$x = 40$ units/ml

$\dfrac{1000 \text{ units/hour}}{40 \text{ units/ml/solution}}$

$\dfrac{1000}{40} : : 1 \times \dfrac{1000}{40} = x$ ml/min

$\dfrac{1000}{40} = 25$ ml/hour

$\dfrac{60 \text{ microdrops}}{60 \text{ minutes}} \times 25 \text{ ml/hour} = \text{microdrops/min}$

$\dfrac{60}{60} \times \dfrac{25}{1} = 1 \times 25 = 25$ microdrops/min

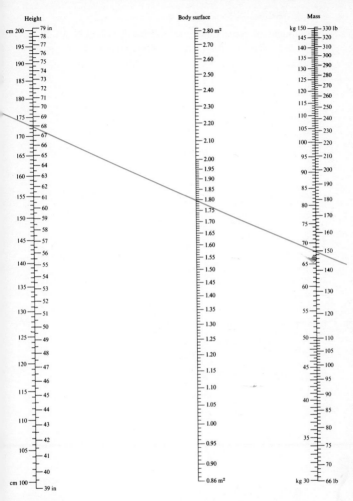

Figure 4-1

Body surface area of adults: nomogram for determination of body surface from height and mass, based on the formula of DuBois and DuBois, Arch Intern Med 17:863, 1916: $S = M^{0.425} \times H^{0.725} \times 71.84$, or $\log S = \log M \times 0.425 + \log H \times 0.725 + 1.8564$ (S: body surface in cm^2, M: mass in kg, H: height in cm).

Courtesy CIBA-GEIGY, Ltd, Basel, Switzerland.

BSA Requirements

The dosages of some drugs are calculated proportionally to the BSA of the patient. BSA is calculated in square meters (m^2). A nomogram is used to correlate height (cm/in) with weight (kg/lb) to determine BSA in square meters (m^2) (Figure 4-1). The drug dose is then ordered mg/m^2.

> Height—68 inches   Equation 10
>
> Weight—150 pounds
>
> $m^2 = 1.80$ BSA
>
> Dose 75 mg/m^2
>
> $1.80 \times 75 = x$ dose
>
> $x = 135$ mg dose

Drug Dose Calculations—Pediatric

There are several methods for calculating pediatric dosage based on age, weight, or BSA. The usual means of calculating pediatric dosage is the milligrams per kilogram method. This method requires conversion of pounds to kilograms before determining the desired dose. Drug literature giving the recommended dose per kilogram/pound of body should be consulted before measuring the desired dose.

Milligrams/Kilogram Body Weight

Convert weight in pounds to kilograms (divide the weight by 2.2):

> Child—22 pounds   Equation 11
>
> Medication—phenytoin 5 mg = 1 kg (child's body weight)
>
> Required dose ___ mg
>
> 1. Convert 22 pounds to kg:
> $22 \div 2.2 = 10$ kg
>
> 2. Determine dose based on 1 kg = 5 mg phenytoin (Dilantin)
>   1 kg (child) = 5 mg (drug)
>   10 kg (child) = x mg (drug)
> 10 kg $\times 5 = 50$ mg
> 50 mg = drug dose

Other Methods

If the dosage is not given in terms of milligrams per kilogram then the pediatric dose is calculated from the standard adult dose. These methods are referred to as rules, and the dosage is calculated by weight in pounds, age in months, age in years, or surface area in square meters compared to an adult dose.

Clark's rule (child of 2 years or more)

This method is based on weight in pounds. The adult dose is multiplied by $\dfrac{\text{wt/lb}}{150\ \text{lb}}$

$$\frac{\text{weight (in pounds)}}{150\ \text{lb}} \times \text{adult dose} = \text{approximate child dose}$$

Equation 12

$$\frac{50\ \text{lb}}{150\ \text{lb}} \times 150\ \text{mg adult dose} = \text{approximate child dose}$$

$$\frac{50}{1} \times \frac{1}{1} = 50\ \text{mg child dose}$$

Fried's rule (infant under 1 year)

This method is based on the age in months. The adult dose is multiplied by the following fraction:

$$\frac{\text{age (in months)}}{150\ \text{months}}$$

(150 months is the age of a 12½-year-old child)

$$\frac{\text{age (in months)}}{150\ \text{months}} \times \text{adult dose} = \text{approximate infant dose}$$

$$\frac{9\ \text{months}}{150\ \text{months}} \times 200\ \text{mg} = \text{infant dose}$$

Equation 13

$$\frac{9}{150} \times \frac{200}{1} = \frac{9}{15} \times \frac{20}{1} = \frac{9}{3} \times \frac{4}{1} = \text{infant dose}$$

$$\frac{9}{3} \times \frac{4}{1} = \frac{36}{3} = 12\ \text{mg infant dose}$$

Young's rule (child of 2 years and older)

This method is based on the age in years of the child. The adult dose is multiplied by the following fraction:

$$\frac{\text{age of child in years}}{\text{age in years} + 12} \times \text{adult dose} = \text{approximate child dose}$$

Adult dose of penicillin 500 mg   Equation 14

Child age—8 years

Child dose = ____ mg

$$\frac{8 \text{ yrs}}{8 \text{ yrs} + 12 \text{ yrs}} \times 500 \text{ mg} = \text{approximate child dose}$$

$$\frac{8}{8 + 12} = \frac{8}{20} = \frac{2}{5} = \frac{500 \text{ mg}}{1}$$

$$\frac{2}{5} \times \frac{500}{1} = \frac{2}{1} \times \frac{100}{1}$$

$$\frac{2}{1} \times \frac{100}{1} = \frac{200}{1} = 200 \text{ mg} = \text{child dose}$$

BSA method

A nomogram is used to correlate the height (cm/in) with the weight (kg/lb) to determine BSA in square meters (m^2) (Figure 4-2). The drug dose is then ordered mg/m^2.

Height—23 inches   Equation 15

Weight—44 pounds

$m^2 = 0.50$ (BSA)

Dose—1 mg/m^2

$0.50 \times 1 \text{ mg} = \text{x dose}$
    $\text{x} = 0.50 \text{ mg drug}$

Other methods using surface area include:

$$\frac{\text{Surface area in square meters}}{1.75} \times \text{adult dose} = \begin{array}{l}\text{approximate}\\ \text{child dose}\end{array}$$

or

$$\frac{\text{Surface area of child}}{\text{Surface area of adult}} \times \text{adult dose} = \text{approximate child dose}$$

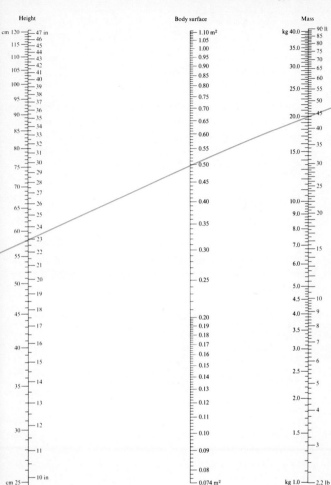

Height

cm 120 — 47 in
      46
115 — 45
      44
110 — 43
      42
105 — 41
      40
100 — 39
      38
95 — 37
      36
90 — 35
      34
85 — 33
      32
80 — 31
      30
75 — 29
70 — 28
      27
65 — 26
      25
60 — 24
      23
55 — 22
      21
50 — 20
      19
45 — 18
      17
40 — 16
      15
35 — 14
      13
30 — 12
      11
      10 in
cm 25

Body surface

1.10 m²
1.05
1.00
0.95
0.90
0.85
0.80
0.75
0.70
0.65
0.60
0.55
0.50
0.45
0.40
0.35
0.30
0.25
0.20
0.19
0.18
0.17
0.16
0.15
0.14
0.13
0.12
0.11
0.10
0.09
0.08
0.074 m²

Mass

kg 40.0 — 90 lb
          85
35.0 — 80
       75
30.0 — 70
       65
25.0 — 60
       55
20.0 — 45
20.0 — 45
       40
15.0 — 35
       30
10.0 — 25
9.0 — 20
8.0
7.0 — 15
6.0
5.0 — 10
4.5
4.0 — 9
3.5 — 8
3.0 — 7
       6
2.5
2.0 — 5
       4
1.5 — 3
kg 1.0 — 2.2 lb

Figure 4-2

Body surface area of children: nomogram for determination of body surface from height and mass, based on the formula of DuBois and DuBois, Arch Intern Med 17:863, 1916: $S = M^{0.425} \times H^{0.725} \times 71.84$, or $\log S = \log M \times 0.425 \times \log H \times 0.725 \times 1.8564$ (S: body surface in cm², M: mass in kg, H: height in cm).

Courtesy CIBA-GEIGY, Ltd, Basel, Switzerland.

IV Fluids

The body's fluid and electrolyte needs are altered by a variety of diseases and conditions. When an individual is ill, these needs are constantly changing. IV therapy is prescribed to correct deficiencies and achieve balance by supplying maintenance requirements of water and electrolytes and replacing any ongoing losses.

Fluid Balance

Fluid Compartments

Although a small amount of body fluid is transcellular, it is primarily intracellular or extracellular. Intracellular fluid (ICF)—fluid within the cells—accounts for approximately 25 liters of fluid in an average-size adult. Extracellular fluid (ECF) is in the spaces between cells (interstitial space) and in the intravascular fluid or plasma. Approximately 15 liters of fluid is contained in the ECF—12 liters in the interstitial space and 3 liters in the plasma or intravascular space. ECF values are similar to chemistry laboratory reports (Table 5-1).

Approximately two thirds of the total body fluid is in the ICF space, and one third is in the ECF space. Fluids shift from one compartment to the other as the concentration of electrolytes (solutes) is altered in the body. Fluids always move from the compartment with the lowest concentration of solutes to that with the greatest concentration. *Dehydration,* or body fluid loss, leads to *greater* concentration of electrolytes in the *extracellular* compartment. This is treated with the administration of IV fluids. Fluid retention in the ECF compartment is treated with sodium restriction and restriction of fluid amounts.

Losses of ECF may be difficult to assess if the patient has pooling of fluids in the bowel, peritoneum, or intestinal spaces, for example, intestinal obstruction, peritonitis, hepatic failure, and burns. These areas are sometimes referred to as a "third space." Surgical patients usually manifest reabsorption after third spacing

Table 5-1   Comparison of electrolyte values for ICF, ECF, and serum values on laboratory reports

Electrolytes	ICF	ECF	Normal Laboratory
Sodium	2-10 mEq/L	138-142 mEq/L	135-145 mEq/L
Potassium	135-155 mEq/L	3.8-5 mEq/L	3.5-5 mEq/L
Chloride	4-10 mEq/L	92-105 mEq/L	100-110 mEq/L
Calcium	<1 mg/dl	<5 mg/dl	8.5-10.5 mg/dl
Magnesium	80 mg/dl	1-2 mg/dl	1.7-3.4 mg/dl

by an increased urine output 48 to 72 hours after the operation. This can often be anticipated, and fluids are adjusted accordingly. As fluid from the third space is reabsorbed into the circulation, the patient is monitored for fluid overload.

Clinical Alert: Headache and confusion may indicate ICF volume changes. Thirst and nausea may indicate ECF volume changes. Noninvasive assessments of plasma volume include examining jugular veins, checking pulse rate, and measuring blood pressure.

Water Balance

Water is essential for life; people can live several weeks without food but only a few days without water. Water maintains blood volume, regulates temperature, transports electrolytes and nutrients to and from cells, and is a part of many biological reactions. Chemically, water and electrolytes work in concert to maintain water balance. Water intake is regulated through the sensation of thirst; water and electrolytes are continuously lost and replaced. Water balance is maintained primarily by the kidneys responding to the concentration of solutes present in the filtered body water.

Actual body water content depends on such variables as age, sex, body composition, and disease processes. Adults are composed of approximately 60% water, and infants of approximately 77%. Women have a slightly lower water content than men because of a larger amount of body fat. There is an inverse relationship between body water and adipose tissue (fat): the more adipose tissue, the less body water. Many disease processes alter body water, for example, renal failure, congestive heart failure, and gastrointestinal dysfunction. These abnormal conditions alter the concentration of electrolytes present in the ICF and ECF and cause a shift in fluid between compartments.

Table 5-2   Normal fluid intake and loss in an adult eating 2500 calories per day (approximate figures)

Intake		Output	
Route	Amount of Gain (ml)	Route	Amount of Loss (ml)
Water in food	1000	Skin	500
Water from oxidation	300	Lungs	350
Water as liquid	1200	Feces	150
		Kidney	1500
TOTAL	2500	TOTAL	2500

From Phipps WJ, Long BC, and Woods NF: Medical-surgical nursing: concepts and clinical practice, ed 3, St Louis, 1986, The C.V. Mosby Co.

Water balance is monitored through body weight. An otherwise unexplained weight change of 1 kg (2.2 pounds) represents a gain or loss of 1 liter of body water. An individual's average daily water intake and water output is approximately 2500 ml (Table 5-2).

Electrolyte Balance

Attaining and maintaining electrolyte balance are critical components of IV therapy, since imbalances can be fatal. Electrolytes are related to at least four fundamental physiological processes: water distribution in the ICF and ECF, neuromuscular irritability, acid-base balance, and maintenance of osmotic pressure.[*] IV therapy is directed at restoring lost electrolytes; once the electrolytes are replaced, the metabolic acid-base balance corrects itself. There are respiratory acid-base disturbances that cannot be corrected with IV therapy alone, such as hyperventilation causing an increased pH secondary to blowing off CO_2 or hypoventilation with CO_2 retention resulting in decreased pH or acidosis. The electrolytes of greatest importance in fluid therapy are discussed below.

[*]Osmotic pressure refers to the pull or force created by random movements in a compartment or area. Fluids always flow from areas of greater concentration to areas of lesser concentration. Concentration in the blood plasma is largely determined by serum proteins, for example, albumin. The osmotic influence (osmolality) of an IV fluid is a key consideration when determining which type of IV fluid to administer in a particular situation.

Sodium

More than any other electrolyte, sodium influences the distribution of body water. Because sodium attracts water, it is the primary factor determining the volume of extracellular space. Sodium is administered intravenously as sodium chloride. Sodium disorders are considered extracellular volume disorders. High sodium concentrations in the plasma (hypernatremia) result from conditions such as an impaired sense of thirst, hyperventilation, fever, head injuries, decreased secretion of antidiuretic hormone (ADH), diabetes insipidus, and the inability of the kidneys to respond to ADH.

Low sodium concentrations in the plasma (hyponatremia) involve an increase in the proportion of water to salt in the blood and result from a disturbance in the ADH secretory mechanism, for example, head injury and severe physiological and psychological stress (this disturbance is called SIADH—syndrome of inappropriate ADH secretion). Hyponatremia may also occur when hypotonic fluids are given to such patients at a time when ADH secretion is excessive.

Hypernatremia	Hyponatremia
Serum sodium > 145 mEq/L	Serum sodium < 135 mEq/L
Hypotension	Hypertension, increased intracranial pressure
Hypervolemia	Hypovolemia
Dry mucous membranes	Increased salivation
Urine volume <30 ml/hour	Low urine specific gravity
Altered mental status	Altered mental status
Coma and death	Coma and death

Clinical Alert: Hypernatremia is corrected slowly—over 48 hours or more—since rapid treatment can produce serious consequences, including loss of consciousness and death. Use normal saline to correct hypernatremia, since normal saline is less concentrated than the serum of a patient with severe hypernatremia. Administer hypertonic sodium chloride solutions 3% to 5% to correct severe hyponatremia and follow with diuretics that will result in the loss of more water than sodium. Instill these solutions cautiously while monitoring closely both neurological and cardiovascular status.

acidosis drives pot. from the cells
K

Potassium

Potassium—the major electrolyte of the ICF—is required to maintain osmotic balance and cell membrane electrical potential and to move glucose into the cell. Plasma potassium, or the potassium found in the ECF and measured by laboratory testing, is influenced by dehydration, blood pH, dietary intake, and diuretic therapy. When potassium balance between the ICF and ECF is altered, cellular metabolism is affected along with the cardiovascular, renal, respiratory, and neuromuscular systems.

Elevated serum potassium levels are referred to as hyperkalemia; reduced serum potassium levels are called hypokalemia. Acidosis drives potassium out of cells, resulting in hyperkalemia; alkalosis drives potassium into cells, resulting in hypokalemia.

Hyperkalemia	Hypokalemia
Serum $K^+ > 5$ mEq/L	Serum $K^+ < 3.5$ mEq/L
Conduction disorders of heart	Ectopic cardiac activity
ECG: peaked T-wave, widened QRS, lengthened P-R	ECG: Flattened T-wave, depressed ST segment
Diarrhea, abdominal pain	Decreased bowel sounds, ileus
Neuromuscular irritability	Muscle weakness, paresthesias
Oliguria or anuria *decreased of urine*	Polyuria *increase of urine*
Cardiac failure	Digitalis toxicity

Potassium is administered intravenously as potassium chloride. Hypokalemia is treated with oral or IV administration of potassium chloride (KCl). A potassium deficit is slowly corrected to avoid development of transient hyperkalemia. Treatment of hyperkalemia depends on the rate at which the potassium level increased. Immediate treatment measures may include IV administration of calcium gluconate, sodium bicarbonate, glucose, or insulin. In mild states of hyperkalemia, oral and IV intake of potassium is restricted.

Clinical Alert:

1. Urine output of at least 30 ml/hr should be verified before beginning IV potassium administration.
2. If the administration rate exceeds 20 mEq/hr, cardiac monitoring is suggested.
3. Potassium should never be administered directly in a concen-

trated form by IV push because of the danger of cardiac arrest.
4. KCl should be thoroughly mixed when adding to an IV bag to prevent layering of potassium at the bottom of the bag.
5. A low dose of lidocaine may be added to the KCl solution to diminish the burning sensation patients complain frequently of when IV infusions contain potassium greater than 40 mEq/L.

Chloride

Chloride is the major electrolyte in the ECF. Chloride levels in blood are passively related to those of sodium, so that when serum sodium increases, chloride also increases. Factors causing losses or gains of chloride frequently affect sodium levels. Increased chloride levels are caused by dehydration, renal failure, or acidosis. Decreased chloride levels result from fluid losses in the gastrointestinal tract (nausea, vomiting, diarrhea, and gastric suction).

Chloride Excess	Chloride Deficit
Serum Cl$^-$ > 110 mEq/L	Serum Cl$^-$ < 100 mEq/L
Dehydration	Fever
Hyperventilation	Nausea and vomiting
Urine output less than 30 ml/hr	Tissue wasting (burns)

Chloride is always administered intravenously in conjunction with sodium and potassium.

Calcium

Calcium, the most abundant electrolyte in the human body, is stored primarily in the skeleton. Greater than 99% of skeletal calcium is unavailable for day-to-day electrolyte regulation. Calcium is present in the blood in two forms: free, ionized calcium that is circulating, and calcium that is bound to protein. The bound form attaches to the plasma protein (albumin) and other complex substances such as phosphates. For this reason it is important to correlate serum calcium concentration with the serum albumin level.

Calcium levels have an effect on neuromuscular function, cardiac status, and bone formation. Disturbances in calcium balance result from alterations in bone metabolism, secretion of parathy-

must be given with chloride

roid hormone, renal dysfunction, and altered dietary intake.

Hypercalcemia	Hypocalcemia
Serum $Ca^{++} > 10.5$ mEq/L	Serum $Ca^{++} < 8.5$ mEq/L
Decreased mental alertness	Neuromuscular irritability, for example, numbness and tingling, hyperactive reflexes, and seizures
Abdominal pain, muscle weakness, nausea and vomiting, and hypertension	Bone pain

Acute symptoms of hypocalcemia are treated with IV administration of calcium gluconate or calcium chloride. Oral calcium supplements are used for chronic hypocalcemic states.

Hypercalcemia treatment includes supportive measures to lower the serum calcium level and to correct the underlying cause. Sodium chloride infusion and the administration of thiazide diuretics, usually furosemide (Lasix), are given to enhance the body's excretion of calcium. IV administration of calcitonin and mithramycin may be given to inhibit bone resorption in bone destructive conditions.

Magnesium

Magnesium is normally obtained from dietary intake. Excretion of magnesium is through the kidneys. Hypomagnesemia is far more common than hypermagnesemia. Conditions associated with magnesium deficits include prolonged malnutrition or starvation, alcoholism, and long-term IV therapy without magnesium supplementation. Symptoms are potentiated by hypocalcemia. Hypermagnesemia occurs most often in patients with renal failure and those with diabetic ketoacidosis, and in those who use excessive amounts of antacids or laxatives.

Magnesium Excess	Magnesium Deficit
Serum $Mg^{++} > 3.4$ mEq/L	Serum $Mg^{++} < 1.7$ mEq/L
Lethargy	Disorentation
Absent deep tendon reflexes	Hyperactive reflexes
Hypotension	Tremors, tetany
Depressed respirations	

Magnesium sulfate solutions can be administered intravenously to correct deficits, although monitoring is required to avoid cardiac effects. Magnesium excess may be treated with the IV administration of calcium gluconate, which reverses the action of magnesium. Glucose or insulin may be given to enhance the renal excretion of magnesium.

Fluid and Electrolyte Loss

The major components of body fluids are water and electrolytes. Water losses occur when water leaves the body through the kidneys, lungs, skin, and gastrointestinal tract. Kidneys are the organs principally responsible for regulating the volume and concentration of all body fluids. When given optimal amounts of water and electrolytes, a normally functioning kidney can maintain water and electrolyte balance. However, during serious illness the kidneys are sometimes unable to make the final adjustments for fluid and electrolyte balance.

Water loss from the lungs and skin increases with elevated temperatures in the environment, fever, rapid respiratory rate, and a loss of skin covering. Examples of situations resulting in skin covering loss are surgical procedures, burns, and wounds. Gastrointestinal losses increase when vomiting and diarrhea are present. Fluid and electrolyte losses are replaced through the intake of food and water.

Assessments and Findings of Fluid and Electrolyte Balance

Assessments	Findings
Compare total fluid intake and total fluid output	Intake should be approximately the same as output
Compare daily weight obtained at approximately the same time on the same scale	A gain of 1 kg of body weight corresponds to 1 liter of fluid
Review serum electrolyte laboratory values	*Fluid excess:* Electrolyte level is diluted, thus laboratory values are decreased *Fluid deficit:* Electrolyte levels are concentrated, resulting in increased laboratory values *Continued.*

Assessments	Findings
Observe clinical status	Condition of mucous membranes, skin, heart rate, presence of thirst, and mental alertness

IV Fluids

IV fluids are classified as isotonic, hypotonic, or hypertonic solutions depending on the effect a fluid has on the ICF and ECF compartments (Table 5-3).

Table 5-3   IV fluids

Fluid and Tonicity	Comments
Saline Solutions	
0.33% Sodium chloride Hypotonic	Extremely hypotonic, used only with close observation
	Does not supply calories
0.45% Sodium chloride Hypotonic	Does not supply calories
0.9% Sodium chloride Isotonic *to replace*	Used to expand plasma volume; provides sodium and chloride in excess of plasma levels; given primarily with blood transfusions and to replace large sodium losses, for example, burns, gastrointestinal fluid loss
	Does not supply calories
3% Sodium chloride Hypertonic	Correction of severe sodium depletion
	Does not supply calories
5% Sodium chloride Hypertonic	Maximum daily amount not to exceed 400 ml; can result in fluid volume excess and pulmonary edema
	Does not supply calories

dextrose do not replace electrolytes
dextrose 5%. 170 calories per liter
10% 340 calories per liter

Table 5-3 IV fluids—cont'd

Fluid and Tonicity	Comments
Dextrose in Water Solutions	
5% Dextrose in water Isotonic	Used to maintain fluid intake or to reestablish plasma volume; does not replace electrolyte deficits; aids in renal excretion of solutes Supplies 170 calories/liter
10% Dextrose in water Hypertonic	Used for peripheral nutrition Supplies 340 calories/liter
20% Dextrose in water Hypertonic	Irritating to veins; acts as a diuretic; may increase fluid loss; central line required Supplies 680 calories/liter
50% Dextrose in water Hypertonic	Must be given through a central line Supplies 1700 calories/liter
70% Dextrose in water Hypertonic	Used to provide calories to persons with compromised renal and cardiac status; central line required Supplies 2400 calories/liter
Dextrose in Water and Saline Solutions	
5% Dextrose and 0.2% NaCl Isotonic	Supplies 170 calories/liter
5% Dextrose and 0.3% NaCl Isotonic	Supplies 170 calories/liter
5% Dextrose and 0.45% NaCl Hypertonic	Used to treat hypovolemia and to promote diuresis in dehydration; used to maintain fluid intake; maintenance fluid of choice if no electrolyte abnormalities Supplies 170 calories/liter
5% Dextrose and 0.9% NaCl Hypertonic	Supplies 170 calories/liter
10% Dextrose and 0.9% NaCl Hypertonic	Supplies 340 calories/liter

50 % 1700 calories

Continued.

Table 5-3   IV fluids—cont'd

Fluid and Tonicity	Comments
Multiple Electrolyte Solutions	
Ringer's solution Isotonic	Electrolyte concentrations of sodium, potassium, calcium, and chloride are similar to normal plasma levels Supplies calories only when mixed with dextrose
Lactated Ringer's solution Isotonic	Electrolyte concentrations similar to plasma levels; lactate for correction of metabolic acidosis; used to replace fluid losses due to bile drainage, diarrhea, and burns; fluid of choice for acute blood loss replacement Does not supply calories
5% Dextrose and lactated Ringer's solution Hypertonic	Used to replace gastric fluid losses; not to be given with blood products Supplies 170 calories/liter
5% Dextrose and electrolyte #2 Hypertonic	Electrolyte maintenance solution Supplies 170 calories/liter

Isotonic Solutions

Isotonic solutions are used to expand ECF volume. These solutions contain the same concentration of solute to fluid as that in body fluid and exert the same osmotic pressure as ECF in a normal, steady state.

Normal saline, or 0.9% NS, lactated Ringer's solution, and 5% dextrose and water all function as isotonic solutions. If an isotonic solution is infused into the intravascular system, fluid volume increases. One liter of isotonic solution expands the ECF by 1 liter. Three liters of isotonic fluid is required to replace 1 liter of blood loss.

Hypotonic Solutions

Hypotonic solutions exert less osmotic pressure than the ECF. Infusion of excessive hypotonic fluids can lead to intravascular fluid depletion, hypotension, cellular edema, and cell damage. Since these solutions can cause serious complications, the patient and the infusion should be monitored closely. The hypotonic solutions of 0.45% sodium chloride and 0.3% sodium chloride provide free water, sodium, and chloride to aid the kidneys in the excretion of solutes.

Clinical Alert: Never administer sterile distilled water intravenously except when using it as a drug diluent, since plain distilled water has an extremely hypotonic effect on red blood cells and can lead to lysis of the red blood cells.

Hypertonic Solutions

Hypertonic solutions exert greater osmotic pressure than ECF. These solutions are used to shift ECF into the blood plasma by diffusing fluid from the tissues to equalize the solutes in the plasma. Rapid administration of a hypertonic solution can cause circulatory overload and dehydration. Hypertonic IV fluids include 5% dextrose in 0.9% saline, 5% dextrose in lactated Ringer's solution, and dextrose and water solutions of 10% dextrose and greater.

Documentation Recommendations

1. Volume and composition of all administered fluids
2. Fluid intake and output
3. Fluid deficit
   a. Eyes: dry conjunctiva, reduced tearing, sunken appearance
   b. Mouth: dry, sticky mucous membranes; dry, cracked lips
   c. Skin: diminished turgor
   d. Neurological: reduced CNS activity
   e. Cardiac: narrowed pulse pressure, lowered blood pressure
   f. Weight: loss
   g. Other: fever, source and amount of any body fluid loss
4. Fluid excess
   a. Eyes: orbital edema
   b. Skin: warm, moist; edema in dependent areas
   c. Cardiac: bounding pulse, vein distention
   d. Respiratory: dyspnea, crackles, wheezes, increased rate, pulmonary edema

5. Electrolyte imbalance
   a. Sodium excess: record urine volume and patient temperature
   b. Sodium deficit: increased viscosity of saliva, increased urine volume, all mental status changes, and signs and symptoms of increased intracranial pressure, for example, headache and increased blood pressure
   c. Potassium excess: irregular heart rate, diminished urine volume, ECG changes
   d. Potassium deficit: muscle weakness, dysrhythmias.

Nursing Diagnoses

- Fluid volume deficit, related to excessive fluid loss from abnormal routes (vomiting, diarrhea, indwelling tubes), diuretic therapy, burns, trauma, and surgical procedures
- Fluid volume deficit, related to inability to receive or absorb fluids, for example, hypermetabolic states (fever), head injury, coma, and electrolyte imbalance
- Fluid volume excess related to excess fluid or sodium intake

Patient/Family Teaching for Self-Management

- Stress that IV fluids do not provide sufficient calories to meet basic energy needs, and when indicated, encourage small, frequent meals.
- Teach signs and symptoms of fluid excess and deficit, for example, significance of weight gain, edema, shortness of breath, dyspnea on exertion, and recognition of gastrointestinal losses.
- Teach measurement of fluid intake and output so patients and family members can participate in record keeping.

Home Care Considerations

Successful home infusion therapy depends on patient motivation, disease stability, and the availability of venous access. A capable person must be present in the home during the infusion to monitor patient changes.

- Instruct patients and caregivers to monitor weight gains and losses and to report significant findings.

- Reinforce the need to report all abnormal findings to the physician, for example, shortness of breath, dyspnea on exertion, edema, elevated temperature; discuss an emergency plan with the patient and caregiver.
- Monitor electrolyte status on a planned basis; ideally, electrolytes should be obtained within 24 hours of initiating infusion therapy; obtain results of recent blood urea nitrogen (BUN), creatinine, blood glucose values, and any other tests relevant to the patient's condition.
- Plan oral fluid and electrolyte supplements with the physician.
- Clearly document all education provided.

Pediatric Considerations

- The smaller the child is, the less fluid there is in each body compartment, especially the ICF.
- Children become dehydrated more quickly than adults and need to have losses replaced more quickly.
- Weigh diapers before and after changes to facilitate accurate measurement of output; replace losses volume-for-volume with a hypotonic electrolyte solution.
- For children under 1 year of age, assess for the presence of a depressed anterior fontanelle and creases on the soles of the feet when dehydration is suspected.
- Weigh children daily while they are receiving IV fluids; consider weighing neonates every 8 hours.
- Assess and document level of consciousness; include tone of cry.
- Infants who are not receiving oral fluids need to have their sucking urge satisfied by pacifiers.

Chapter
Resources

Evaluation for Fluid Imbalance

Assessments	Findings
Blood pressure	*Fluid deficit:* Fall in systolic blood pressure (BP), decreased pulse pressure, and postural hypotension
	Fluid excess: Increased BP, no postural changes
Pulse	*Fluid deficit:* Weak, thready pulse
	Fluid excess: Bounding pulse; increased pulse rate; tachycardia may be present with *either* fluid *excess* or *deficit*
Jugular vein	*Fluid deficit:* Flat neck veins
	Fluid excess: Vein distention visible, pulsation higher than 2 cm above sternal angle when head of bed raised 45 degrees
Respirations	*Fluid deficit:* Rare crackles and wheezes; dry, thick secretions
	Fluid excess: Crackles and wheezes; moist secretions
Edema	*Fluid deficit:* Infrequent edema
	Fluid excess: First found in dependent parts, for example, sacral edema in persons on bed rest; pedal edema in ambulatory persons
Skin turgor	*Fluid deficit:* Loose, toneless skin; skin tense when lifted with two fingers; inaccurate assessment in elderly
	Fluid excess: Good skin turgor

Evaluation for Fluid Imbalance—cont'd

Assessments	Findings
Intake and output	*Fluid deficit:* Output greater than intake; slow urine output; high specific gravity
	Fluid excess: Intake greater than output; rapid urine output; low specific gravity
Weight	*Fluid deficit:* Weight loss
	Fluid excess: Weight gain

Clinical Alert: Major alterations in fluid balance can occur before clinical signs and symptoms are present. Approximately 3 days following major abdominal surgery, fluid can move rapidly from the abdominal cavity and interstitial space to the intravascular compartment, creating fluid overload. Expect significant change in the patient's output at this time.

IV Medication Administration

6

More medications are being administered intravenously than before, and nurses are assuming greater responsibilities related to IV medication administration. With increased usage has come a greater understanding of the benefits and risks of this treatment modality. Many technical improvements have been made in equipment, and innovative and time-saving measures have been developed to increase the efficacy of this practice. This chapter addresses principles of IV medication administration, methods of delivering drugs intravenously, and information on select drugs.

General Principles

Indications for IV Drug Administration

IV drug administration is beneficial for several reasons:
1. Assurance that effective concentrations of the drug are achieved rapidly
2. Control over onset of peak serum drug concentrations
3. Production of a biological effect when a drug cannot be absorbed by the oral route.
4. Drug administration to patients who are unable to take oral medications

Drug Dose Calculations

Since drugs for IV medication administration are injected directly into the vascular system, IV doses are often lower than those administered through other routes. Although the doses of many drugs administered intravenously are calculated according to the patient's weight, doses are adjusted also according to drug distribution and the patient's absorption ability, metabolism, and excretion.

Serum albumin levels are important to drug distribution, since drugs bind to receptor sites on plasma proteins (especially albumin) and tissues. Since only a drug that is not bound to a plasma protein or to a tissue is able to exert a therapeutic effect, patients with *low* serum albumin levels have *more* adverse effects. This occurs because more free (unbound) drug is available to exert a therapeutic effect. Drug binding influences both drug effectiveness and the duration of the effect.

Drug metabolism and excretion are the two components involved in drug elimination from the body. Metabolism refers to the transformation of the drug to a water-soluble form that allows excretion to occur. Patient age and underlying disease affect elimination. Elderly people usually have diminished liver and kidney function and less muscle mass than younger persons. Any disease process that alters hepatic or renal function also can cause a prolonged drug effect.

A drug's half-life is defined as the time required for plasma levels of the drug to fall to half of the original level. Drug half-life is influenced by both metabolism and excretion rates. In addition, the half-life determines the frequency of doses that must be administered to maintain a steady drug state. Some drugs, such as heparin, must be administered continuously to effectively maintain blood levels. However, antibiotics, and various other drugs may be given intermittently. When a new drug is given, loading doses are frequently required to reach therapeutic plasma concentrations rapidly.

Clinical Alert: Because the kidney and the liver are the major organs involved in drug excretion, the half-life of a drug is extended in patients with renal or liver disease and in the elderly.

Combination Drug Therapy

Combination therapy refers to intended drug interactions. Drugs are often administered in combination to potentiate a desired effect that is enhanced by the interaction of two or more drugs; for example, meperidine (Demerol) and promethazine (Phenergan) are often administered together to enhance sedation and postoperative pain control. Metabolism, excretion, and binding can all be affected when multiple drugs are administered.

Complications of IV Drug Administration

Every complication that may develop with IV therapy is present when drugs are administered intravenously, including infiltration, phlebitis, and the potential for embolism or infection. Adverse or unplanned effects such as diminished drug potency and toxicities can occur often when multiple drugs are administered. Mild adverse effects are called side effects; serious adverse effects are called toxicities.

Almost any drug is capable of producing a hypersensitivity (allergic) reaction. Hypersensitivity reactions often occur more quickly when drugs are administered intravenously than when given orally. When the IV system is used for more than one purpose, for example, fluid administration and medication administration, interaction and incompatibilites develop more often.

Hypersensitivity reactions

Hypersensitivity reactions can range from a mild skin rash to anaphylaxis. The onset of the reaction is usually sudden, although reactions can be delayed as much as 30 to 60 minutes. Usually, the faster the reaction is, the more severe it will be. Although any drug can cause an adverse reaction, drugs that most commonly cause hypersensitivity reactions are antimicrobials—especially penicillins and amphotericin B, dextran, dyes used for diagnostic testing, and some chemotherapy drugs, particularly L-asparaginase.

The extent of the reaction is related to the amount of drug administered and the patient's degree of hypersensitivity. Skin reactions—sudden onset of inflammation and itching—are the most common and can be treated symptomatically with antihistamines. Signs and symptoms of anaphylaxis include respiratory distress (wheezing and cyanosis), skin reactions (itching, blotchy, skin wheals), and symptoms of circulatory collapse (rapidly falling blood pressure, weakness, thready pulse, and dizziness). Gastrointestinal symptoms—nausea, vomiting, and diarrhea—occur less frequently. Suffocation resulting from laryngeal edema is the most common cause of death following an anaphylactic reaction. The following steps should be taken when any reaction is identified:

1. Stop the medication immediately.
2. Keep an IV line open.
3. Observe the patient's respiratory status; if the patient has respiratory difficulty, keep him in an upright position if possible while summoning help.
4. Notify the physician.
5. Prepare to administer emergency medications.
6. Monitor vital signs.

7. Begin resuscitation if a respiratory or cardiopulmonary arrest occurs.

Clinical Alert: Epinephrine (Adrenalin) followed by diphenhydramine (Benadryl) are the drugs of choice for treating anaphylaxis. Other drugs that may be given include hydrocortisone (Solu-Cortef) and aminophylline (Theophylline).

Drug incompatibility

Information on drug compatibilities is complex and changes frequently as administration systems and solutions change. New research and additional experience result in changes in drug treatment recommendations. Because of conflicting literature and the complexities involved with compatibility information, absolute statements are difficult to make. Compatibility is most influenced by pH. Drugs with similar pH are compatible; those with significantly different pH are incompatible and should not be administered together. Although compatibility charts are helpful tools, they should be used judiciously, since conflicting information is often presented as a result of varied study conditions.

Incompatibility occurs when either two drugs or a drug and an IV solution are mixed to make a product that is unsuitable for safe administration. Physical, chemical, and therapeutic changes in the drug result from incompatibility. These changes result in loss of drug activity, unexpected adverse reactions, precipitate formation, and adverse clinical changes in the patient such as anaphylaxis, multiple pulmonary infarctions, and platelet aggregation.

Physical changes in the drug are the most common and the easiest to detect visually. These may be a change in color or precipitate formation. A precipitate formation is often determined by the concentration of the drug, the pH of the solutions, the sequence of additives, and the amount of standing time since admixture. Precipitation can occur immediately, hours later in the tubing or filter, or in the IV catheter, thus causing occlusion. Visual inspection cannot detect very small precipitates.

Chemical changes result in irreversible drug degradation. The product resulting from chemical change is less active than expected, and therefore the therapeutic effect is altered.

Therapeutic changes occur when two or more drugs combine to produce an effect that is pharmacologically antagonistic or synergistic, an effect usually considered adverse.

IV Drug Administration Rate

The IV drug administration rate is determined by the amount of drug that can be given over 1 minute. When the administration rate is not known, an IV medication should be administered at the rate of 1 mg/min.

Methods of IV Medication Administration

IV drugs may be given using a variety of techniques. The method chosen depends on the desired effect and the available supplies and equipment. When selecting a method, the following variables that can affect serum levels of drugs should be considered: flow rate, location of injection site, drug volume, and fluid volume of the tubing. Descriptions of various methods follow.

IV Push

High concentrations of medication are administered directly into an IV lock or through an injection port to achieve rapid and predictable serum levels. The IV injection is usually given over 5 minutes or less. This method of drug administration is designed to administer bolus doses.

1. Procedure
   a. Insert the syringe with medication into the IV lock or through an injection port as close to the IV cannula as possible after cleansing the port with an alcohol swab.
   b. Clamp off the primary IV line (if applicable).
   c. Administer the drug at prescribed rate.
   d. Use a second syringe to administer flush solution.
   e. If the medication bolus was given directly into an IV lock, flush the lock with 2 to 3 mls of normal saline or heparinized saline according to policy; continue exerting pressure on the syringe while withdrawing it to prevent a backflow of blood into the IV catheter.
2. Advantages
   a. The drug response is rapid and predictable; this method is frequently used in emergency situations.
   b. The nurse is able to observe the patient throughout the procedure.
3. Disadvantages
   a. Adverse effects can be expected at the same time and rate as therapeutic effects.

b. The IV push method has the greatest risk of adverse effects and toxicity, since serum drug concentrations are sharply elevated.

Clinical Alert: Flush IV tubing after administering a drug to ensure that the complete dose is delivered; otherwise a portion of the drug may remain in the port or may layer in the IV tubing. Administer the flush at the same rate as the medication bolus, since the flush pushes medication from the tubing into the patient's vein.

IV Piggyback

IV piggyback is a type of intermittent drug infusion. IV medication is diluted in a small bag or syringe of D5W or normal saline and administered as a drip over approximately 30 minutes. The administration time varies according to the volume of solution intended for infusion.

1. Procedure
   a. Spike medication container with an IV administration set.
   b. Hang the medication container at or above the level of the primary IV (Figure 6-1).
   c. The drug may be administered simultaneously with a compatible IV fluid; if the fluid entering the IV cannula is not compatible with the medication, flush the line with 2 to 3 ml of normal saline before beginning medication infusion and stop the flow of the main solution; if the primary infusion cannot be interrupted, consider using a dual-lumen catheter or administering the medication through a second site as an intermittent infusion.
   d. Infuse the drug at prescribed rate.
   e. Following drug administration, the secondary set may remain attached to the IV set or removed until the next dose; if the line is removed, cap the end of the line with a new needle.
2. Advantages
   a. Incompatibilities are avoided.
   b. A larger drug dose can be given at a lower concentration per milliliter than would be practical with the IV push method.
3. Disadvantages
   a. Administration rate is not controlled precisely unless the infusion is electronically monitored.

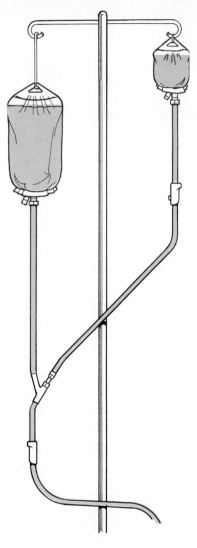

Figure 6-1
Piggyback IV medications.

b. IV set changes can result in the wasting of a drug assumed to have been given.

c. Bags are available with only D5W and normal saline solutions.

d. The added volume of 50 to 100 ml of IV fluid can cause fluid overload in some patients.

Intermittent Infusion

The drug is prepared in the same manner as an IV piggyback solution. Instead of a secondary IV line being attached to the existing infusion, an intermittent infusion is attached directly to an IV lock.

1. Procedure
   a. Flush IV lock with 2 to 3 ml of normal saline.
   b. Insert the infusion into the IV lock and secure the junction with tape.
   c. Infuse the drug at the prescribed rate.
   d. Following drug administration, flush the lock with normal saline or heparinized saline solution; exert a positive pressure on the syringe when withdrawing from the IV lock to prevent a backflow of blood into the IV catheter.

2. Advantages and disadvantages are the same as for the piggyback method.

Volumetric Chamber

Medication is added to the volume control chamber and diluted with IV fluid. Infusion is generally over 15 minutes to 1 hour (Figure 6-2).

1. Procedure
   a. Add medication to the chamber.
   b. Add the required amount of IV fluid.
   c. Infuse the drug at the prescribed rate.
   d. Following completion of the drug infusion, resume the IV infusion or flush the IV lock.

2. Advantages
   a. Runaway infusions are avoided without the use of electronic equipment.

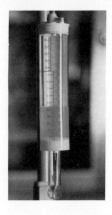

Figure 6-2
Volumetric chamber.   *Buretrol*
From Perry AG and Potter PA: Clinical nursing skills and techniques, St Louis, 1986, The CV Mosby Co.

    b. Volume of fluid in which the drug is diluted can be adjusted easily.

  3. Disadvantages

    a. The drug must travel a long distance before it reaches the patient; there is a significant time delay during very slow infusion rates before the drug dose reaches the patient.

    b. When the chamber empties and the infusion is slowed, a large amount of the drug can remain in the IV tubing.

    c. Incompatibilities may develop when the chamber is used for multiple drugs.

    d. It is necessary to change the labeling on the chamber each time a new solution is added.

Continuous Infusion

Medication is added to a large volume of parenteral solution and administered continuously. These infusions are usually regulated with an IV pump or controller to ensure an accurate flow rate (Figure 6-3).

1. Procedure
   a. Place time-tape on bag, even when a pump or controller is used, to verify administration rate.
   b. Spike the IV container with an IV administration set.
   c. Regulate flow rate.
   d. Observe the patient at least every hour during the infusion; many medications require more frequent patient monitoring.
2. Advantages
   a. Admixture and bag changes can be performed every 8 to 24 hours.
   b. Constant serum levels of the drug are maintained
3. Disadvantages
   a. When not monitored electronically, there is an imprecise control over the administration rate.
   b. Drug compatibility problems may develop if the line is used to administer piggyback or IV push medications.

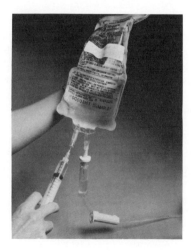

Figure 6-3
Injecting medications into IV solution.
From Perry AG and Potter PA: Clinical nursing skills and techniques, St Louis, 1986, The CV Mosby Co.

Clinical Alert: Inadequate drug mixing can result in serious and undesired drug effects. To ensure adequate mixing of any drug added to an IV solution, do not add a medication to a hanging bag and follow these guidelines:

1. Use a long needle—at least 1 inch in length—to inject drugs into the bag; otherwise a concentration of the drug may remain in the port.
2. To assist with mixing, use force when injecting a medication.
3. Agitate or rotate the bag several times to aid in mixing the drug with the IV solution.

If the drug added is not as dense as the IV solution, the medication floats to the top of the solution; if the drug is more dense than the IV solution, it remains at the bottom of the container. Incomplete mixing of any drug results in drug delivery that is not consistent. Aminophylline is a drug that is less dense than most IV solutions; potassium chloride is more dense that most IV solutions.

Retrograde Administration

Retrograde administration is used primarily with infants and small children. The retrograde system allows for drug administration for over 30 minutes without increasing the IV flow rate. The medication is administered away from the patient with a special IV set (Figure 6-4).

1. Procedure
   a. Obtain special Benzing administration set.
   b. Administer the drug against the flow of the IV fluid.
   c. Displace an equal volume of IV maintenance solution and discard this solution.
   d. Resume the prescribed IV flow rate.
2. Advantages
   a. Does not add to the fluid intake of patients with restricted fluid intake.
   b. Minimal drug loss in the IV system.
3. Disadvantages
   a. Drugs may be administered at an unpredictable rate if low-volume IV tubing is not used.
   b. Problems with drug interactions can develop when more than one medication is administered through the system.

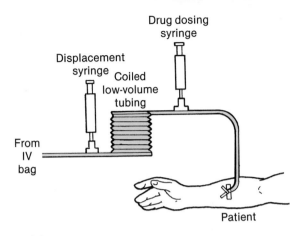

Figure 6-4
Retrograde drug administration.

Clinical Alert: Adding extension tubing to an IV set can significantly increase the time it takes the medication to reach the patient, especially at slow flow rates.

Special Drug Manufacturer Packaging

Many innovative premixed and partially mixed medications are available from drug manufacturers. These packages allow medications to be admixed in their original packaging at the time of administration. Use of these medications is convenient and reduces wastage and labor costs. The major disadvantage associated with special packaging is an increase in cost per dose. Consult the manufacturer's directions for procedures related to administration.

Use of Electronic Pumps and Controllers

IV pumps and controllers are designed to regulate flow rates precisely and are used widely with medicated IVs. Fluids are delivered automatically at a preselected rate, and many record the amount of fluid infused, automatically prime tubings, and offer prompts to assist with pinpointing infusion problems. Most machines are accurate within 2% of the selected rate. They vary according to ease of use, pressure-monitoring capabilities, size, programmability, microrate-infusion capability, need for special tubings, battery life, availability of printouts, and method of operating. Most pumps may be used for IV, arterial, and epidural drug infusions. The manufacturer's recommendations for specific device features always should be checked.

IV Controllers

Controllers deliver fluids with the aid of gravity. The IV fluid container must be placed approximately 36 inches above the IV site to overcome venous resistance and operate properly. A photoelectric eye monitors the flow rate. Controllers are designed to sound an alarm when resistance is detected and thus are useful for the detection of infiltrations.

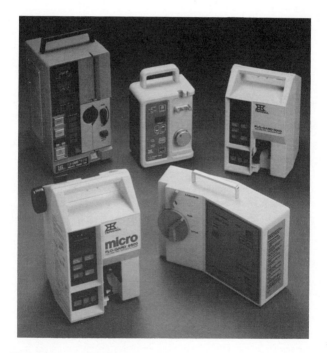

Figure 6-5
Flo-Gard infusion pumps.
Manufactured by Baxter Healthcare Corp, Deerfield, Ill.

IV Pumps

Pumps provide pressure to fluid delivery when it is necessary to overcome filter resistance, viscous solutions, small-gauge catheters, and patient activity (Figure 6-5). When the pump senses resistance, it attempts to maintain the IV flow rate by increasing the pressure of fluid delivery. Select features of IV pumps and related comments follow.

Features	Comments
Operating mechanism	Operate with a diaphragm, piston (syringe), or peristaltic mechanism
Pressure	The maximum pressure applied before an occlusion alarm sounds varies; some pumps allow variable settings according to the desired applications (IV, arterial, epidural)
Programmability	Allows portions of the total daily dose to be given at desired times, rates, and intervals; usually able to accommodate at least a 24-hour drug supply for ambulatory patients
Bolus doses	Pumps designed for patient-controlled analgesia administration have the capacity to deliver bolus doses of drug on demand
Flow rate	Can range from 0.1 to 2000 ml/hr according to machine selected
Variable pressure	Variable pressure settings allow solutions of different viscosity to be administered
Multiple infusions	One to four solutions may be regulated at different rates by one machine; some have piggyback options
Alarms	Alarm conditions can include occlusion, machine malfunction, empty container, air in line, door open, and low battery; the number of safety alarms varies according to model
Tamper-proof settings	Desirable especially for use with children and with narcotic infusions

Continued.

Features	Comments
Size	Wide range of sizes available; ambulatory pumps are designed specifically to deliver small volumes of 50 to 100 ml; the pump and a bag are worn by the patient to allow mobility; may have a piston or peristaltic action
Cost	Wide range according to features; dedicated tubing costs also vary widely according to the manufacturer

Considerations When Working With Pumps and Controllers

1. Fill the administration set's drip chamber to the fill line or half full to allow the sensor to monitor the drip accurately; most drip sensors are placed at the top of the chamber.
2. Most tubing cassettes should be inverted for priming.
3. Verify accurate functioning at regular intervals.
4. Always follow manufacturer's directions.
5. Do not use tubing clamps with a pump or controller.

V. Imp.

Avoiding Medication Errors

As in the administration of all medications, the potential for error is a concern. This concern is particularly serious in IV administration because of the rapid flow rate. To minimize the risk of errors, always follow the five "rights" of medication administration: right drug, right dose, right patient, right time, right route. In addition, observe the following precautions:

1. Always read the label on all drugs and verify the medication(s) with the physician's order before administration.
2. Resolve questions about unfamiliar drugs before administration; know the expected dosage ranges, administration rates, incompatibilities, adverse effects and antidotes, and the intended usages of the drugs.
3. Clarify ambiguous medication orders; encourage the use of only approved abbreviations in physician orders.
4. Consider the possibility of drug interactions and take appropriate precautions.
5. If a patient has had an allergic reaction in the past, be cau-

tious especially when a new drug is added; when starting a new drug, particularly an antibiotic of the same type as one the patient has been allergic to in the past, question the possibility of another reaction.

6. Before administering a drug, check the patient's armband and record for the presence of allergies.

7. Verify dosage calculations with another person to avoid mathematical errors; when possible, refer to calculation tables for medications frequently administered.

8. Chart medications immediately after administration to avoid the possibility of administering a repeat dose.

9. To the extent possible, reconstitute drugs so that they can be administered at a rate of 1 mg/min.

10. Encourage the implementation of standardized IV drug dilutions to simplify administration rate calculations.

Select Drug Information

Antimicrobial Agents

Antibiotic, antifungal, and antiviral agents are frequently administered intravenously. These drugs may be administered prophylactically to decrease the incidence of infection after certain operations, empirically to initiate therapy directed against the most likely infecting organism before receipt of culture and sensitivity reports, or therapeutically. Therapeutic coverage is achieved based on culture and sensitivity reports. Antibiotics act either by inhibiting bacterial cell wall synthesis and producing a defective cell wall, or by altering intracellular function of the bacteria, for example, electron transport, target DNA binding. The categories of antimicrobial agents most widely used are discussed below.

Cephalosporins

Cephalosporins are widely used, relatively safe antibiotics. There is a wide dosage range between toxic drug levels and subtherapeutic drug levels. Adverse effects are similar to those of penicillins; approximately 3% to 5% of individuals who have adverse reactions to penicillin have adverse reactions to cephalosporins. Those who have had anaphylaxis are most susceptible to an allergic reaction with a cephalosporin. Adverse effects may include hypersensitivity, phlebitis, diarrhea, neutropenia, and altered liver function.

Aminoglycosides are chemically inactivated by cephalosporins. The following target organisms are affected by cephalosporins:

1. First generation: Most gram-positive organisms and some gram-negative organisms.
2. Second generation: Increased gram-negative action, decreased gram-positive effectiveness.
3. Third generation: Expanded gram-negative coverage, decreased gram-positive coverage.

Aminoglycosides

Aminoglycosides are used most often to treat bacteremia, systemic infections, and urinary tract infections. IV administration is always used to achieve a systemic effect, since the drugs are not absorbed from the gastrointestinal tract. Target organisms include gram-negative aerobes, staphylococci, and mycobacteria. The mechanism of action is interference with bacterial protein synthesis and replication.

One of the major differences among the various aminoglycosides is toxicity incidence. Adverse effects are a concern when using aminoglycosides because of the narrow range between therapeutic and toxic effects. To monitor drug dosages closely, periodic drug peak and trough levels are drawn. Trough levels are measured before administration of a subsequent dose, and peak levels are drawn within 30 minutes of the completion of a dose. Trough levels greater than 2 μg are associated with increased toxicities (see Table 6-1 for a listing of some IV drug peak and trough levels). Adverse effects of aminoglycosides include the following:

1. Nephrotoxicity. Persons who already have diminished renal function are particularly at risk for developing this effect; when other nephrotoxic drugs are administered, this effect is potentiated.
2. Ototoxicity. Tinnitus, loss of high-frequency hearing, and altered balance may all result from ototoxicity.
3. Neuromuscular blockade. Respiratory depression or paralysis can occur in conjunction with anesthetics.

Table 6-1   Serum drug level monitoring

Drug	Trough	Peak
Aminoglycosides (gentamicin, tobramycin, amikacin)	Within one-half-hour of next dose Serum level: <2 μg/ml	One-half-hour after end of 30-minute infusion, or 15 minutes after end of 1 hour infusion Serum level: 5 to 10 μg/ml
Vancomycin	Within one-half-hour of next dose Serum level: <10 μg/ml	1 hour after end of infusion Serum level: 20 to 40 μg/ml
Digoxin-IV	5 to 24 hours after last dose, just before next dose preferred Serum level: 0.8 to 2 μg/ml	Do not draw
Aminophylline	Just before dose Serum level: 10 to 20 μg/ml	1 hour after dose Serum level: 10 to 20 μg/ml
Dilantin-IV	Just prior to dose Serum level: 10 to 20 μg/ml	One-half-hour after end of infusion

Penicillins

Penicillins act by inhibiting bacterial cell wall synthesis. Most gram-positive organisms and some gram-negative cocci are sensitive to penicillins. Adverse effects can include cutaneous reactions, gastrointestinal symptoms, especially diarrhea, hypersensitive reactions, and renal damage (see Table 6-2 for a listing of cephalosporins, aminoglycosides, and penicillins).

Table 6-2   Aminoglycosides, cephalosporins, and penicillins

	Generic Name	Trade Name
Aminoglycosides	Amikacin	Amikin
	Gentamicin	Garamycin
	Kanamycin	Kantrex, Klebcil
	Neomycin	Neomycin
	Netilmicin	Netromycin
	Streptomycin	Streptomycin
	Tobramycin	Nebcin
Cephalosporins		
First Generation	Cefazolin	Ancef, Kefzol
	Cephalothin	Keflin, Seffin
	Cephapirin	Cefadyl
	Cephradine	Velosef
Second Generation	Cefamandole	Mandol
	Cefonocid	Monocid
	Ceforanide	Precef
	Cefoxitin	Mefoxin
	Cefuroxime	Zinacef
Third Generation	Cefoperazone	Cefobid
	Cefotaxime	Claforan
	Ceftazidime	Fortaz, Tazidime
	Ceftizoxime	Cefizox
	Ceftriaxone	Rocephin
	Moxalactam	Moxam
Penicillins		
Natural Penicillins	Penicillin G	Pentids
	Penicillin V	Pen V, V-Cillin
Aminopenicillins	Amoxicillin	Amoxil, Larotid, Polymox, Sumox, Trimox
	Ampicillin	Omnipen, Polycillin, Principen, Supen, Totacillin
	Bacampicillin	Spectrobid
	Cyclacillin	Cyclapen
	Hetacillin	Versapen
Extended Spectrum Penicillins	Azlocillin	Azlin
	Carbenicillin (oral only)	Geocillin

Table 6-2   Aminoglycosides, cephalosporins, and penicillins—
cont'd

	Generic Name	Trade Name
Extended Spectrum Penicillins	Mezlocillin	Mezlin
	Piperacillin	Pipracil
	Ticarcillin	Ticar
Penicillinase-Resistant	Cloxacillin	Tegopen
	Dicloxacillin	Dynapen, Pathocil
	Methicillin	Staphcillin
	Nafcillin	Nafcil, Nallpen, Unipen
	Oxacillin	Bactocill Prostaphilin

Amphotericin B

Amphotericin B is the most widely used antifungal drug. The method of action is injury of the cell wall of the fungi. This drug is not effective against other organisms. Because of the toxicities and side effects associated with administration of amphotericin B, it is used to treat only serious fungal infections that are progressive in nature and potentially fatal. Before treatment a fungal infection diagnosis is positively established through culture or histology studies. Therapeutic levels remain in the body up to 20 hours after each infusion, since the drug is excreted very slowly through the urine.

Because this medication is infused as a suspension, the drug should *not* be filtered during administration but should be administered slowly, usually over 2 to 6 hours. No other medications should be piggybacked with amphotericin B because of its incompatibility with most drugs.

Patients experience many side effects during administration of this drug including shaking chills and fever, nausea and vomiting, and muscle and joint pains. For this reason patients are started on reduced doses of the drug, and the dosage is increased in increments until desired levels are reached. Baseline vital signs should be taken before initiation of an infusion so that the effect of the adverse effects can be assessed more accurately. To alleviate some of the unpleasant side effects experienced with this drug, patients are often premedicated with diphenhydramine, hydrocortisone, and analgesics. A summary of adverse reactions reported in conjunction with amphotericin B follows.

System	Adverse Reactions
Central nervous	Headache, vertigo, convulsions
Cardiovascular	Cardiac toxicity, hypertension, hypotension
Gastrointestinal	Anorexia,* weight loss,* nausea,* vomiting,* diarrhea*
Hematologic	Anemia,* phlebitis,* thrombocytopenia, leukopenia
Musculoskeletal	Muscle and joint pains*
Renal	Compromised renal function*; monitor BUN and serum creatinine levels
General	Blurred vision, tinnitus, fever with shaking chills, rash, anaphylaxis, potassium depletion*

*Most common effects.

Aminophylline

Aminophylline is used as a bronchodilator to symptomatically treat asthma and bronchospasms that may occur with chronic bronchitis and emphysema when oral and inhalant drugs are insufficient. The drug is distributed rapidly throughout the ECF and body tissue within 1 hour following initiation of therapy. Metabolism occurs mainly in the liver, and excretion is through the kidneys.

If a patient has not been receiving oral theophylline, a loading dose of aminophylline is usually administered as a bolus before initiating an infusion to reach therapeutic dosage rapidly. Aminophylline infusions should be regulated by an IV pump or controller, since the administration rate is the dominant factor causing toxicities. Following is a summary of adverse reactions to aminophylline.

System	Adverse Reactions
Central nervous	Headache, insomnia, anxiety, confusion, restlessness, seizures
Cardiovascular	Hypotension, palpitations, fast or slow heart rates
Gastrointestinal	Anorexia, nausea and vomiting, abdominal cramps

System	Adverse Reactions
Renal	Albuminuria
Respiratory	Tachypnea
General	Hyperglycemia

(Refer to *Chapter Resources* for aminophylline infusion rates.)

Heparin

Heparin is an anticoagulant used for the treatment of all types of thromboses, emboli, and some coagulopathies such as disseminated intravascular coagulation. In addition, heparin is used to treat patients undergoing certain types of major surgery or requiring prolonged immobilization. The effects of heparin are immediate and predictable. Heparin combines with other factors in the blood to inhibit the conversion of prothrombin to thrombin and fibrinogen to fibrin. The duration of action is from 4 to 6 hours, and the plasma half-life averages 1 to 2 hours. IV heparin may be given intermittently every 4 to 6 hours as an IV bolus or as a full-dose infusion over several days. Adverse reactions to heparin are listed below.

System	Adverse Effects
Hematologic	Hemorrhage, reversible thrombocytopenia, rebound hyperlipidemia
Integumentary	Urticaria, transient hair loss
Renal	Hematuria, increased loss of sodium, suppression of renal function
Respiratory	Asthma
General	Chills, fever, anaphylaxis

(Refer to *Chapter Resources* for heparin infusion rates.)

Narcotic Infusions

Although narcotics may be administered intravenously for severe pain as a bolus dose, the most effective analgesia is achieved when a consistent serum level of narcotic is maintained. IV narcotic administration allows predictable drug absorption through the use of an infusion that is titrated to achieve analgesia, or with a specialized, programmable pump that allows the patient to administer predetermined doses of the narcotic. The latter method is called patient-controlled analgesia, or PCA (Figure 6-6).

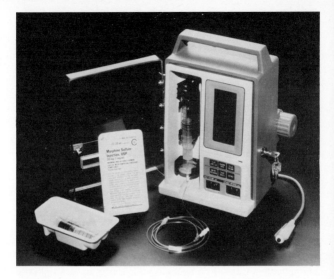

Figure 6-6
Patient-controlled analgesia (PCA).
Courtesy Abbott Laboratories, Abbott Park, Ill.

Narcotic infusions are usually prepared as large-volume solutions and are regulated by a pump or controller to ensure accurate drug delivery. Patients require frequent monitoring for respiratory depression and the presence of other adverse narcotic effects such as nausea and vomiting. (Refer to *Chapter Resources* for morphine infusion rates.)

PCA doses are individualized for the patient and allow the patient to deliver a drug dose as needed for pain relief by pushing a button connected to the PCA pump. Frequently, patients use less medication than they are allowed and have accelerated recoveries following surgical procedures: the more consistent pain control is, the greater ease of movement the patient experiences. PCA pumps are used with an existing IV line that infuses at a rate of at least 30 ml/hour to maintain patency of the IV catheter between drug doses. To be eligible for PCA, patients should be mentally alert and receptive to learning PCA operation. Patients should also be able to understand and follow directions and should not have a history of drug or alcohol abuse.

Successful PCA requires clear patient instruction. The patient should receive a complete explanation of the pump and an explanation of the lockout interval before surgery. Periodic doses of narcotic may be administered by the nurse when the patient is sleeping to allow prolonged rest periods.

PCA pumps are designed with safeguards, for example, allowed doses and lockout intervals, to protect against tampering and misuse of the drugs. Physician orders for PCA include:

1. Drug to be administered—usually morphine or meperidine (Demerol)
2. Dose volume—the amount administered each time the PCA infusor is activated
3. Time lockout interval—the period during which the pump cannot be activated and no analgesia can be delivered; this allows time for the dose to take effect before the patient receives another; the usual lockout interval is 6 to 10 minutes for postoperative pain, but it may be longer according to patient need.
4. Volume limits—the maximum volume to be delivered over a prescribed period of time

Epidural narcotic infusions are used increasingly for the management of acute and chronic pain (Figure 6-7). The discovery of opiate receptors and endorphins has led to the use of morphine in

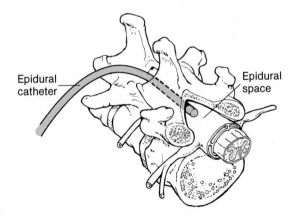

Epidural catheter   Epidural space

Figure 6-7
Epidural space with epidural catheter.

the epidural space for pain control. Opiates such as morphine have a direct spinal effect, acting at receptor sites in the dorsal horn of the spinal cord. The major mechanisms by which morphine is thought to gain entry to the dorsal horn are through diffusion into and across the cerebrospinal fluid and through venous entry along a nerve root sleeve. Epidural narcotics provide site-specific pain relief with relatively low morphine doses.

There are three different systems used to deliver morphine to the epidural space. The first system is a totally internal system in which an epidural catheter is connected to a reservoir placed in the abdomen. This reservoir's mechanism allows slow, continuous administration of morphine. It must be filled with the desired drug concentration on a weekly or biweekly interval by inserting a Huber needle into the reservoir septum. This system is permanently placed and used most often for the patient requiring long-term pain management.

In the second system, an epidural implantable port with a catheter connected to the portal chamber is anchored to muscle tissue over a bony surface. The catheter is tunneled subcutaneously and then threaded into the epidural space at the desired level, usually L1 or L2. A Huber needle is used to access the septum of the portal chamber, and medication is pumped continuously with an ambulatory, programmable pump. Like the first system, this system is permanently placed and used for the patient who requires long-term pain management.

The third system consists of an externally threaded catheter that is tunneled subcutaneously from the epidural space to an abdominal exit site. It is then connected to an injection cap and a 0.22 μm filter with extension tubing through which morphine can be administered intermittently by an IV infusion pump. This system may be used on a temporary or a permanent basis. Temporary catheters are placed for pain relief following operative procedures such as thoracic, abdominal, orthopedic, and vascular surgery. Temporary catheters may be used also to evaluate the efficacy of this treatment modality before placing a permanent catheter for the management of chronic pain.

Epidural morphine must be free of preservatives and additives and should be prepared under a laminar flow hood. Commercially prepared morphine is available in the following concentrations: 1 mg/ml, 2 mg/ml, 5 mg/ml, and 25 mg/ml. Many of the ambulatory infusion pumps can hold a 100 ml infusion bag that allows bag changes every 4 to 5 days for patients who receive epidural infusions for chronic pain management (Figure 6-8).

Adverse effects associated with epidural morphine include respiratory depression, urinary retention, pruritus, and nausea and vomiting. These effects are encountered most often with postoperative use of epidural analgesia and may be reversed by an IV naloxone (Narcan) infusion. Patients require ongoing monitoring for pain relief, sedation level, and adverse drug effects, especially respiratory depression. As with all catheters, the site should be assessed for pain or tenderness.

Clinical Alert: Patients receiving epidural narcotic infusions require ongoing observation of their blood pressure and pulse and respiratory rates. Crucial times when the drug will have the most potent effect on the respiration are during the first 2 hours following catheter insertion and again after 6 hours.

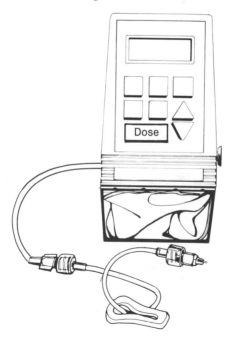

Figure 6-8
CADD-1® ambulatory infusion pump.
Courtesy Pharmacia Deltec Inc, St Paul, Minn.

Use *preservative-* and *additive-free* morphine for epidural analgesia; never administer IV solutions by the epidural route.

Check catheter placement before injecting a drug by aspirating for clear fluid with bubbles. If yellow- or blood-tinged fluid is aspirated, *stop* the procedure and notify the physician, since only clear fluid should be aspirated. Expect to feel some resistance as the medication is injected.

Documentation Recommendations

- Observation of the site before and after infusion or injection of a drug
- Medication name, dose, route, and time of administration
- All supplies used for medication administration
- Name and amount of all flush solutions (normal saline or heparin)
- Any patient complaints of discomfort symptoms experienced in conjunction with the medication; record actions taken to alleviate symptoms and report to physician when applicable
- When using narcotic infusions, document pain relief status, sedation levels, analgesia level, and respiratory rate; when using PCA, record the total dose delivered since the last notation and the number of doses delivered

Nursing Diagnoses

- Infection, potential for, related to a break in sterile technique during drug preparation or administration
- Injury, potential for, related to adverse effect of medication
- Comfort, altered: pain, related to infiltration or phlebitis

Patient/Family Teaching for Self-Management

Education for home IV medication administration is most effective when a standardized content is developed and a standardized approach is taken to patient teaching. Each skill requires a demonstration and a return demonstration by the patient or the responsible caregiver. Materials sent home with the patient for reference need to be easy to read and should contain pictures of all procedures for nonreaders.

Hospital-based teaching for self-medication administration

should include the following information:

- Name, dose, and frequency of the drug to be administered
- Aseptic technique
- Use and disposal of needles and syringes
- How to obtain medications and other supplies
- Medication storage requirements and medication preparation (if applicable)
- How to administer the drug
- Infusion pump operation (if applicable)
- Expectations for medical follow-up, for example, physician visit, laboratory sampling
- Adverse drug effects and what should be done if these occur
- The importance of strict compliance with the medication regimen and how to recognize symptoms of a worsening condition
- Care of the IV access including problem recognition and troubleshooting techniques

Home Care Considerations

I. Home teaching
  A. Information taught in the hospital should be reviewed in the home.
  B. The patient should demonstrate each self-care skill to the nurse.
  C. Inspect storage areas for adequacy.
  D. Teach acceptable thawing methods when frozen drugs are used (NOTE: microwaves are *not* recommended for thawing antibiotics in the home).

II. Documentation recommendations
  A. Initial visit
    1. Record a detailed physical assessment of the patient, including manual dexterity and coordination.
    2. Document information on home adequacy and safety in relation to IV therapy.
    3. Assess and record the patient or caregiver's ability to comply with the prescribed regime; include specific situations that indicate evidence of understanding.
    4. Inform the patient of 24-hour staff accessibility and when use of the emergency department is indicated.

B. Ongoing visits
   1. Record treatment compliance including storage of supplies; check the temperature of the home refrigerator if temperature is an important factor in drug stability.
   2. Evaluate and record the patient's response to the prescribed treatment noting any adverse effects and the corrective action taken; include an assessment of vital signs and a review of equipment operation.
   3. Provide evidence of the review of appropriate laboratory data.
   4. Document all other care given.
   5. Record the periodic treatment review conducted with the patient's physician.
C. Dismissal visit
   1. Detail the assessment leading to termination of therapy.
   2. Record all discharge instructions.
III. Quality assurance issues for home IV medication administration—periodic audits should be conducted on topics that indicate safety and availability of all appropriate services; some items include:
   A. All educational topics were taught and documented.
   B. There is timely delivery of medications, supplies, and equipment.
   C. Medication information was provided to the patient.
   D. There is 24-hour availability of professional staff for problem solving.
   E. All nursing care providers have current certification for resuscitation, for example, Basic Cardiac Life Support.
   F. When IV antibiotics are administered, there is documentation of infection by culture and sensitivity results; the patient is medically stable before home administration has begun; and there is evidence of acceptable infection cure rates in the home setting (it is desirable for a pharmacist to be available to provide pharmacokinetic dosages and drug information).

Pediatric Considerations

■ Children are especially susceptible to drug and fluid overload; use as little fluid as possible to dilute medications and to flush the lines of critically ill infants.

- Use low-volume tubing to assist in controlling the amount of fluid administered to a child and to help predict accurately when the drug effect can be expected.

- Knowledge of body weight in kilograms is essential for correct drug calculation.

- Observe and document the IV system frequently—at least every 30 minutes to 1 hour.

- Use preservative-free saline for flushing the IV systems of neonates.

- Ideally, electronic pumps and controllers used with toddlers and children should include tamper-proof features.

- Microinfusion pumps are preferred for use with neonates; these pumps can infuse fluids in increments of 0.1 ml/h, thus providing delivery of potent drugs at precise rates.

Chapter
Resources

Many medications administered by continuous IV infusion require calculations involving several steps. To minimize these calculations, conversion charts are provided in the following boxes:

Aminophylline Infusion Rate
1000 ml solution with 1000 mg Aminophylline
Concentration (1mg/ml)

Volume	Infusion Rate (ml)	Mg/Hr
1000 ml	5	5
	10	10
	15	15
	20	20
	25	25
	30	30
	40	40
	50	50
	60	60

Heparin Infusion Rate
500 ml solution with 20,000 units Heparin
Concentration (40 units/ml)

Volume	Infusion Rate (ml)	Units/Hr
500 ml	5	200
	10	400
	15	600
	20	800
	25	1000
	30	1200
	35	1400
	40	1600
	45	1800
	50	2000
	55	2200
	60	2400

Morphine Infusion Rate
500 ml solution with 100 mg Morphine Sulfate
Concentration (1 mg/5 ml)

Volume	Infusion Rate (ml)	Mg/Hr
500 ml	5	1
	10	2
	15	3
	20	4
	25	5
	30	6
	35	7
	40	8
	45	9
	50	10
	55	11
	60	12

Parenteral Drug Administration Audit

	Yes	No	NA

Critical Elements

1. Checks medication orders with physician orders
2. Verifies that the medication matches the patient for whom it is ordered
3. Verifies that the patient is not allergic to medication
4. Administers medication in:
   a. Prescribed dose
   b. Prescribed time
   c. Prescribed route
5. Documents:
   a. Name of medication
   b. Dose
   c. Route
   d. Time
   e. Your name or initial, according to policy
   f. Response of the patient to the medication if indicated
   g. Patient education regarding potential side effects of drugs
   h. Blood return status and frequency

Routes of Drug Administration

1. IV Push Medications:
   a. Checks IV site for infiltration and patency
   b. Administers medication without introducing contaminate
   c. Administers IV at prescribed rate
   d. Validates blood return before, during, and at the end of drug administration (when administering chemotherapy)
   e. Following IV push medication, locks the IV catheter according to agency policy
2. IV Piggyback Medications:
   a. Checks IV site for infiltration/patency

Parenteral Drug Administration Audit—cont'd

	Yes	No	NA
b. Administers medication without introducing contaminate			
c. Administers IV at prescribed infusion rate			
d. Administers IV drug with prescribed dilution			
e. Flushes IV site in a timely manner following completion of infusion to ensure site patency			
3. Continuous IV Infusions:			
a. Checks IV site for infiltration/patency			
b. Administers medication without introducing contaminate			
c. Administers IV at prescribed rate			
d. Uses electronic-controlled devices to monitor and assist in administration of drug infusion			
e. Attaches time-taped label to IV solution			
f. Following completion of IV continuous infusion, locks IV catheter or discontinues peripheral IV site			
4. Intraperitoneal (IP):			
a. Checks IP site for patency			
b. Administers medication without introducing contaminate			
c. Administers IP drug at prescribed rate			
d. Following completion of drug administration, injects normal saline to maintain catheter patency			
5. Intraarterial (IA):			
a. Checks IA site for patency			
b. Administers medication without introducing contaminate			
c. Administers IA drug at prescribed rate			
d. Electronic pump is used to monitor and assist in drug administration			
e. Validates blood return q2hr with continuous IV			

Continued.

Parenteral Drug Administration Audit—cont'd

	Yes	No	NA
f. Following completion of IA drug, injects normal saline or heparinized saline to maintain catheter patency			
6. Intrathecal:			
a. Prepares drug in 3 ml syringe and attaches 23-gauge butterfly needle with tubing to syringe			
b. *Physician* injects drug via Ommaya reservoir or lumbar puncture			
c. Following completion of intrathecal drug, the *physician* flushes device with preservative-free saline			
Management of Drug Extravasation of Antineoplastic Agents			
1. Can state signs and symptoms of drug extravasation			
2. Can state the procedure for drug extravasation			
3. Knows placement of supplies used in management of drug extravasation			

TOPICS FOR POLICY STATEMENTS CONCERNING IV INSTRUMENTATION

Indications for Use of Pumps or Controllers

1. Priority list for use during high patient census
2. Administration of medications including
   a. Statement regarding intermittent medications and heparin locks
   b. Central lines
   c. Arterial lines
   d. Special applications, for example, double- or triple-lumen catheters, blood
   e. Administration of chemotherapy and treatment of infiltration (extravasation) of chemotherapeutic drugs
   f. Registering central venous pressure measurement

 3. Tracking of accumulated volumes
 4. Inspection of site when using an infusion pump
 5. Pressure titrations
 6. Use of volume limit feature
 7. Transfer of patients, that is, unit-to-unit
 8. Use of volumetric sets (burettes)
 9. Responsibilities of users including registered nurses, licensed practical nurses, nurse's aides, ancillaries
10. Documentation of instrument use on patient record
11. Special sets required

Blood and Blood Component Administration

7

General Principles of Blood Transfusion Therapy

Blood transfusions have been a major factor in restoring and maintaining quality of life for patients with cancer, hematological disorders, and trauma-related injuries and those who have undergone major surgical procedures. Although blood transfusions are significant for the return to homeostasis, they can be detrimental. Many complications can result from blood component therapy, for example, potentially lethal acute hemolytic reactions, transmission of infectious disease (hepatitis, AIDS), and febrile reactions. Most life-threatening transfusion reactions result from incorrect identification of patients or inaccurate labeling of blood samples or blood components leading to the administration of incompatible blood. Monitoring patients receiving blood and blood components and administration of these products are nursing responsibilities. Blood components should be administered by competent, experienced, well-prepared personnel following the guidelines of the accrediting organizations and agencies providing blood component therapy.

Blood Group Antigens, Antibodies, Rh Factor, HLA Typing

Blood is composed of several constituents that play a major role in blood transfusion therapy. These components—antigens, antibodies, Rh factor, and HLA—contribute greatly to the success of any transfusion.

An antigen is a substance that elicits a specific immune response when coming in contact with foreign matter. The body's immune system responds by producing antibodies to destroy the invader. This antigen (Ag) and antibody (AB) reaction is demonstrated by agglutination or hemolysis. The antibody in the serum responds to the invading antigen by clumping the red cells together and rendering them ineffective or by completely destroying the red cell. Blood typing systems are based on Ag-AB reactions that determine blood compatibility.

The ABO blood group (type) is important in transfusion therapy. Blood type is determined by detection of both antigens on the red cells and corresponding antibodies in the plasma. The antigens on the red cells that are important in the ABO system are the A antigen and the B antigen. Individuals with type A blood have A antigen present on red blood cells; type B individuals have B antigen present; and type O individuals have neither antigen present.

Corresponding antibodies exist in the serum for each of the antigens (A, B). These antibodies occur naturally in the system. The antibodies, anti-A and anti-B, act against the antigen normally present. If the patient's ABO blood type is B, the B antigen is present on the red blood cells and the anti-A antibody occurs naturally.

After the ABO system, the Rh factor is the group of red cell antigens with greatest clinical importance. Unlike anti-A and anti-B, which occur in normal, unimmunized individuals, Rh antibodies do not develop without an immunizing stimulus. Persons whose red blood cells possess D are called Rh positive; those whose cells lack D are called Rh negative, no matter what other Rh antigens are present. The presence of this antibody (anti-D) may cause destruction of the transfused cells as in the case of hemolytic disease of the newborn.

Blood typing identifies the ABO and Rh groupings in the donor blood. Cross matching then determines the compatibility of donor and recipient cells. ABO and Rh compatibility criteria are essential in blood transfusion therapy.

The HLA system is the next component to consider in transfusion therapy. It is based on antigens present on leukocytes, platelets, and other cell antigens. HLA typing and cross matching are usually necessary before granulocyte transfusions or repeated platelet transfusions. Granulocytes and platelets with HLA typing compatible with the patient have a longer life span when infused. HLA-matched granulocytes and platelets *usually* are *not* administered to patients who are expected to be candidates for a bone

O. Universal Donor   *A*
                              B
AB Pos.   *AB Neg - rarest - can't recei*

marrow transplant to diminish potential graft-versus-host disease.

Indications for Transfusion

The primary indications for transfusion are to provide adequate blood volume and prevent cardiogenic shock, increase the oxygen-carrying capacity of blood, and replace blood platelets or clotting factors to maintain hemostasis. Numerous blood components are available, each with its own potential benefits and adverse effects.

Whole blood

Transfusing a unit of whole blood (500 ml) over 30 to 60 minutes increases the blood volume by this amount. The four general rules for transfusion of whole blood are as follows:

1. Transfuse whole blood only for the treatment of acute, massive hemorrhage.
2. Do not give whole blood when the ABO is unknown.
3. Use platelet concentrates and fresh frozen plasma to correct impaired hemostasis when large volumes of whole blood have been transfused.
4. Administration of whole blood should be synonymous with multiple transfusions.

Packed red blood cells

Packed red blood cells are the component of choice to restore or maintain oxygen-carrying capacity. Transfusing packed red blood cells increases the oxygen-carrying capacity with minimal expansion of blood volume and therefore is indicated when chronic anemia and congestive heart failure exist.

Leukocyte-poor red blood cells are given to multiparous women and previously transfused patients who develop antibodies to leukocytes or platelets.

Platelet concentrates

Indications for platelet transfusion relate to the platelet count, the functional ability of the patient's platelets, and the patient's clinical condition. Individuals with platelet counts of 20,000/mm^3 or less and do not have specific platelet-destroying disease benefit from prophylactic transfusion. Patients who are actively bleeding or require major surgery require a platelet count of 100,000/mm^3.

Granulocyte transfusion

Only patients with documented granulocyte dysfunction should receive granulocyte transfusion, for example, severe neutropenia with a granulocyte count of less than 500/mm^3 and evidence of significant infection or temperature greater than 38.3° C with lack of responsiveness to antibiotic to which the organism is known to be sensitive. The patient receiving granulocyte transfusions should have a good chance of recovering from the episode of neutropenia. Granulocytes should be transfused as soon as possible after collection but must be infused within 24 hours. The granulocyte concentrates are usually given daily for at least 4 to 6 days unless bone marrow recovers or severe reactions occur.

Febrile reactions often occur in patients receiving granulocyte concentrates. Antipyretics (nonaspirin) are administered for this reaction. Meperidine injection may be prescribed by the physician to stop shaking chills.

Massive transfusion

Massive transfusion is the replacement of at least half of the patient's blood volume at one time or the replacement of the patient's total blood volume within a 24-hour period. A blood volume is estimated as 75 ml/kg or about 5000 ml (10 or more units of whole blood) in a 70 kg adult.

Complications that may result from massive transfusion include circulatory overload, microemboli, hypothermia, citrate toxicity, hyperkalemia, and coagulation disorders. Patients receiving massive transfusions must be observed closely during the transfusion process. Replacement of blood volume requires rapid infusion (greater than 100 ml/min) of *warmed* blood components or isotonic saline solutions. Frequent laboratory testing is performed during and after the transfusion process to monitor critical values—hemoglobin, hematocrit, prothrombin time, platelet count, sodium, potassium, and calcium levels, and arterial blood gases.

Frequently transfused patients

Following frequent transfusions, alloimmunization to red cells, platelets, and leukocyte (HLA) antigens may occur. This results in cross matching difficulty and febrile and allergic reactions. The patient receiving frequent transfusions should be closely monitored throughout the transfusion process. Administration of the blood component is usually given over an increased infusion time.

3 - 4 hrs. + infusion of blood

Quality Control Measures

Blood bank responsibilities

Blood collection facilities have the responsibility for providing the safety and efficacy of each blood product it collects. The American Association of Blood Banks, American Red Cross, and Federal Drug Association provide rules, regulations, and standards for operation to which all blood bank centers must comply.

Criteria for collection of donor blood is composed of the following:

1. Brief health history
2. Screening for diseases (hepatitis, AIDS, and malaria)
3. Check for vital signs (blood pressure, temperature, pulse, and respiration)
4. Minimum age of 17 years
5. Weight not less than 110 pounds
6. Freedom from any skin disease
7. Time since last blood donation at least 56 days
8. Hemoglobin level of at least 12.5 g/dl or higher for females and 13.5 g/dl for males

Procedure for blood collection

To prevent any potential contamination to the blood specimen, a thorough, skilled, sterile procedure is used. The skin is scrubbed with povidone-iodine solution, and the blood is collected into sterile, labeled tubes and bags. The donor's blood is tested for ABO grouping, Rh type, including D, antibody screening, syphilis serology, and hepatitis B and HIV viruses.

To ensure accuracy in collecting blood samples for recipients of transfusions and for those providing blood donation, the following guidelines have been developed:

1. The intended recipient and the blood sample shall be identified positively at the time of the collection.
2. Blood samples shall be obtained in stoppered tubes, each identified with a firmly attached label bearing at least the recipient's first and last names, identification number, and the date.
3. The completed label shall be attached to the tube before leaving the recipient.
4. There must be a mechanism to identify the person who drew the blood.

5. Before a specimen is used for blood typing or compatibility testing, all identification information on the request form shall be confirmed by a qualified person as being in agreement with that on the specimen label; *in case of discrepancy or doubt, another specimen shall be obtained.*

(See *Chapter Resources* for ''Risks and benefits of blood from various sources.'')

Storage techniques

Red cell products are stored under temperature-controlled refrigeration in the range of 1° to 6° C. Platelets are usually stored at 22° to 24° C (room temperature) and require gentle agitation before transfusion. Plasma separated from whole blood shortly after collection can be frozen at $-18°$ C or lower for use as coagulation factor-rich plasma (fresh-frozen plasma).

The blood bank cannot refrigerate and later reissue *any* blood component meant to be stored at 1° to 6° C if the temperature of the component exceeded 10° C (50° F) at any time. This will happen if the blood component is removed from the blood bank refrigerator for longer than 30 minutes.

Clinical Alert: Refrigeration of blood products on the nursing unit does not ensure accurate temperature regulation and is never acceptable.

Release of blood products

Only qualified blood bank personnel may issue any blood component, and only after following all the guidelines for proper identification of the blood unit—ABO grouping, Rh type, antibody screening, and expiration date (Figure 7-1). The ABO and Rh group must match on the donor unit and the requested transfusion form. On some occasions, substitutions occur in the blood bank.

Group O packed red cells (not whole blood) may be substituted for any ABO group. Rh (D) negative red cells may be safely transfused to Rh (D) positive patients. Rh (D) positive red cells may *not* be transfused to Rh (D) negative patients. However, it is acceptable to transfuse Rh (D) positive plasma products to Rh (D) negative patients, since Rh (D) antigens are on the red cells only.

Separation techniques

Pheresis is a process that removes whole blood from the donor and then separates it into component parts by centrifugation, with the

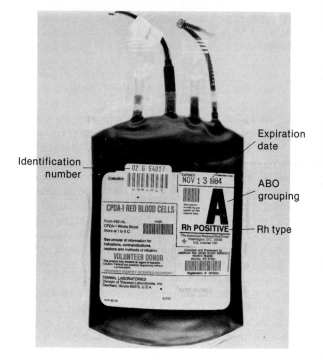

Figure 7-1
Blood product identification.

desired component harvested. The remainder is returned to the donor, thus allowing collection of large amounts of a single component for an individual recipient. This technique is used for selective collection of platelets or white cells (granulocytes), and provides human leukocytes and matched platelets in sufficient numbers of ABO-compatible granulocytes for specific patients.

Cell saver

Cell saver equipment is used to salvage the patient's own blood normally lost during surgery. The blood is collected through a suction device and filtered to remove clots, tissue, and bone fragments. After the blood is washed and rinsed in a saline solution, it is spun in a centrifuge to isolate red blood cells. The red cells are then ready for reinfusion in 5 to 10 minutes. Other blood component therapy may be given in addition to this process to replace blood loss. This method of blood salvage is used for operative procedures requiring 3 or more units of blood for tranfusion. Advantages include the immediate availability of needed blood and the absence of disease transmission or hemolytic, allergic, or febrile reactions. This salvage method minimizes use of blood from blood banks and maximizes patient safety.

Time of blood production administration

Identification of the patient and the proper blood component are the most important procedures in transfusion safety. The correct blood product must be verified, and all labels must be read carefully. All information on the blood product (donor number, ABO group, Rh type, and expiration date) must be compared and matched with the patient's identification bracelet and the transfusion requisition. Discrepancies in spelling, identification numbers, or expiration dates should not exist. All the identification steps must be confirmed by another licensed nursing personnel or blood bank personnel before the transfusion is initiated. Baseline vital signs must be obtained, and the patient must be monitored throughout the transfusion process. On completion of the infusion, the date and time the blood unit was initiated and infusion completed must be documented on the transfusion requisition. Signatures of the personnel confirming all identification information and initiating the transfusion must also be recorded on the requisition.

Equipment and Supplies Used for Transfusions

Equipment

Blood warmers

The warming of blood to the body temperature is necessary during transfusions in certain clinical situations. Research indicates that rapid or massive administration of cold blood has a hypothermic effect on the patient and could have lethal consequences. Patients with potent cold agglutins (unexpected antibodies in the patient's serum that react at temperatures below $20°\,C$) need to have the blood warmed before transfusion to diminish potential adverse effects. Exchange transfusions in neonates and children receiving rapid or massive transfusions must always be warmed, especially when given through a central line. Hypothermia produced by the rapid infusion of cold blood may lead to dysrhythmia and cardiac arrest. For patients requiring extensive operative procedures, a 2° C body temperature loss is not uncommon, reducing the normal body temperature to 35° C. In these situations blood must be infused at this temperature (35° C) to prevent further heat loss.

An effective blood warmer provides a constant temperature

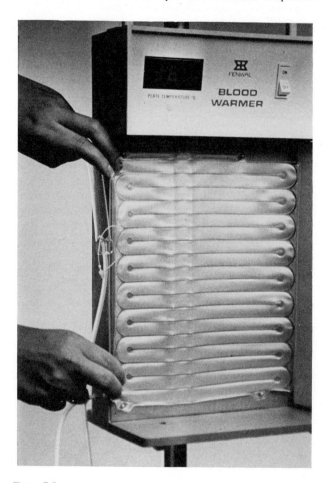

Figure 7-2
Fenwal Blood Warmer.
Manufactured by Baxter Healthcare Corp, Fenwal Division, Deerfield, Ill.

between 32° and 37° C and flows to 150 ml/min. Because warm blood dilates veins, reduced resistance helps to offset flow loss that may result when a warmer is attached. Commercial blood warmers may use a warm bath or dry incubator through which blood passes in sterile, disposable, plastic coils to warm the blood (Figure 7-2). Safety mechanisms include thermostats and alarms for close monitoring of the blood temperature. Follow the prescribed manufacturer's directions for appropriate use and the specific tubings and supplies required (Figure 7-3).

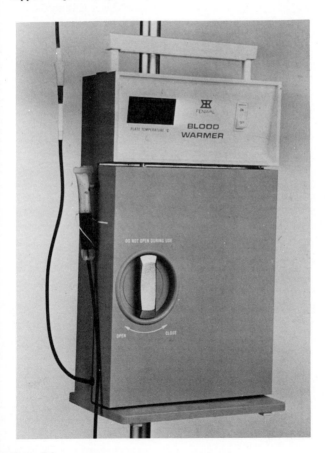

Figure 7-3
Fenwal Blood Warmer.
Manufactured by Baxter Healthcare Corp, Fenwal Division, Deerfield, Ill.

Clinical Alert: Heating blood under hot-water faucets, in incubators, or in microwave ovens can cause hemolysis and is never acceptable.

Pressure cuffs

A pressure cuff is the most commonly used device for increasing the flow rate during transfusion. To increase flow rate, the pressure cuff sleeve is secured snug around the blood bag. The pressure cuff is then filled by a pressure manometer (similiar to a blood pressure cuff) that inflates the sleeve with air. As the blood unit empties, the pressure sleeve decreases. Agency guidelines for use of pressure cuffs should be followed.

Electronic infusion devices

The use of an electronic infusion pump is strongly advised for all pediatric transfusions, although the flow rate is difficult to regulate when small volumes are administered. Gravity flow administration (as used in the adult) is contraindicated because of its potential for allowing too much blood flow over a short period of time. Whenever electronic infusion devices are used, the nurse should be knowledgeable of the features of the device used, for example, alarm operation and rate consistency, rate and volume of infusion, memory, power supply, maintenance, and the manufacturer's recommendations for the types of solutions the device is capable of delivering. Not all electronic infusion devices are acceptable for use in transfusing blood products.

Supplies

Filters

Blood and components must always be transfused through a filter designed to retain blood product debris. Standard filters have a pore size of about 170 μm. To use a blood filter properly, the tubings and filter must be primed adequately. The filter needs to be completely covered with blood or component, and the drip chamber in the tubing should be approximately half full. Incomplete priming can result in air being trapped in the filter, thus causing an inaccurate drop rate. Damage to blood cells may occur if they fall on the exposed filter. Priming procedures differ slightly from one brand of filter and tubing to another; therefore it is important that the manufacturer's instructions included with each set are followed.

Microaggregate filters with a pore size of 20 to 40 μm are used occasionally for massive transfusions, open-heart surgery, and preparation of leukocyte-poor blood. These filters trap the smaller particles that have potential for causing microemboli. For routine blood transfusions, microaggregate filters are used more often with children than with adults. The manufacturer's guidelines for the correct procedure in priming the filter and (if applicable) for flushing the filter after the transfusion should be followed.

Clinical Alert: Do not use a blood filter set for more than four hours. If the flow rate decreases after more than 1 unit has been transfused, you may have to change the filter set.

Tubings

Filtered IV tubings may contain a single line from the blood bag to the patient or a Y-type (dual line). The Y-type set allows the infusion of normal saline while the blood component bags are being initiated or changed. This dual line offers the availability of normal saline to be used as a diluent for packed red blood cells that are too viscous to flow properly. In the event of a blood transfusion reaction, the dual line provides an immediate IV access for isotonic solutions (Figure 7-4).

Only normal saline (0.9% USP) may be administered with blood. Solutions such as 5% dextrose in water or Ringer's lactate solution can cause in vivo hemolysis or initiate coagulation of the donor blood. Medications should *never* be added to a unit of blood.

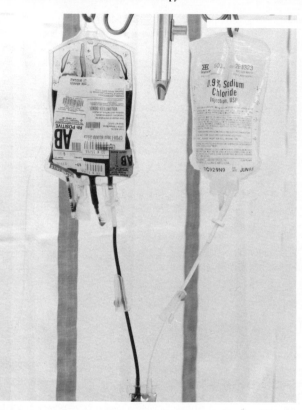

Figure 7-4
Blood administration with normal saline.
From Perry AG and Potter PA: Clinical nursing skills and techniques, St Louis, 1986, The CV Mosby Co.

Blood and Blood Components

Table 7-1 lists many blood and blood components with the approximate volume of each unit, the recommended filter, and the administration rate. The comment section refers to ABO and Rh compatibility and specific product preparation for infusion. The agency blood bank or blood center should be referred to for blood product information.

Text continued on p. 141.

Table 7-1 Blood and blood components

Product	Infusion Guidelines
Packed Red Blood Cells (PRBCs) *Volume* 300 to 350 ml *Filter* Standard blood filter 170 μm or microaggregate filter	Infusion over 1½ to 2 hours; maximum: 4 hr/unit; if blood loss, transfuse as rapidly as the patient can tolerate; if the patient is in unstable cardiovascular balance—chronic severe anemia, congestive heart failure, very small or young—and circulatory overload is a concern, ask blood bank to split unit so administration may be slower than 4-hour maximum *Comments:* Must be ABO and Rh compatible; occasionally Rh_O negative will be transfused to an Rh_O positive patient, but *never* an Rh_O positive to an Rh_O negative; group O packed red cells may be given to *any* blood group, provided the Rh type is appropriate; cross match is required
Washed Red Cells (WRCs) (Leukocyte-poor) *Volume* 200 to 280 ml *Filter* Standard 170 μm blood filter	Infuse over 1½ to 2 hours *Comments:* Same as PRBCs; blood bank requires notification to prepare WRCs; cells expire 24 hours after washing
Frozen-Deglycerolized Red Cells (FDRCs) *Volume* 200 to 250 ml	Infused over 1½ to 2 hours *Comments:* Same as PRBCs; blood bank will not deglycerolize until

Continued.

Table 7-1   Blood and blood components—cont'd

Product	Infusion Guidelines

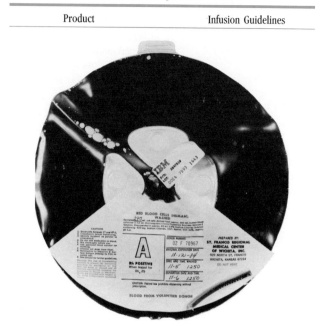

Washed red cells.

FDRCs
Filter
Standard 170 μm blood filter

Comments:
requested; required time to deglycerolize, approximately 1 hour; used primarily for transplant patients or patients who have multiple antibodies; expires 24 hours after deglycerolizing

Whole Blood
Volume
450 to 500 ml
Filter
Standard 170 μm blood filter

Infuse over 2 to 3 hours; maximum: 4 hr/unit
Comments:
Must be ABO and Rh exact

Table 7-1   Blood and blood components—cont'd

Product	Infusion Guidelines
Fresh-Frozen Plasma (FFP) *Volume* 175 to 225 ml *Filter* Special component filter; standard blood filter may be used	Infused over 15 to 20 minutes when given for bleeding or clotting factor replacement; 1 to 2 hours when given for other reasons *Comments:* Must be ABO compatible; Rh_O antigens not in plasma; no cross match required; group AB plasma may be given to any blood group; blood bank does not thaw until required to do so; required time to thaw, 20 minutes; expires 24 hours after thawing
Albumin—25% salt poor *Volume* 12.5 g/50 ml *Filter* Special tubing comes with this product	Infuse within 1 hour *Comments:* Dosage based on BSA requirements (estimating blood and plasma volume); refer to manufacturer's package insert; very hypertonic
Albumin—5% *Volume* 12.5 g/250 ml *Filter* Special tubing comes with this product	Infuse within 1 hour *Comments:* Dosage based on BSA requirements (estimating blood and plasma volume); refer to manufacturer's package insert
Plasma Protein Fraction (PPF) *Volume* Varies according to scheduled dose *Filter* Special tubing comes with this product	Infuse no more than 10 drops/min *Comments:* No typing or cross matching required; used for volume expansion

Continued.

Table 7-1   Blood and blood components—cont'd

Product	Infusion Guidelines
RhO Immune Globulin (RhoGam) *Volume* 1 ml *Filter* None	Given intramuscularly (IM) *Comments:* Usually ordered from blood bank
Immune Serum Globulin *Volume* Up to 1.2 ml/kg body Weight *Filter* None	May be given IV or IM *Comments:* Usually ordered from pharmacy; supplies IgG antibodies
Purified Factor VIII Concentrate (Hemofil, Hyland) *Volume* Freeze-dried Reconstitute with diluent provided *Filter* Filter needle provided with product	Administered intravenously as fast as tolerated by patient to a maximum of 6 ml/min; monitor pulse rate while infusing *Comments:* Use for hemophilia A patient (classical hemophilia or Factor VIII deficiency); usually ordered from pharmacy; preheat diluent to 37° before reconstituting, and use within 3 hours
Purified Factor IX Concentrate (Complex, Hyland) *Volume* Freeze-dried Reconstitute with diluent provided *Filter* Filter needle provided with product	Same as Purified Factor VIII *Comments:* Use for hemophilia B patient (Christmas disease, factor IX deficiency); usually ordered from pharmacy; preheat diluent to 37° before reconstituting and use within 3 hours

Table 7-1   Blood and blood components—cont'd

Product	Infusion Guidelines
Fibrinogen Use cryoprecipitate	*Comments:* Each unit of cryoprecipitate contains approximately 150 mg fibrinogen per 15 ml of plasma
Platelets (Random) *Volume* 60 to 70 ml/unit; minimum order for adult: 6 units;	Administer intravenously as rapidly as patient can tolerate; recommend 150 to 200 ml/hr; may be given more

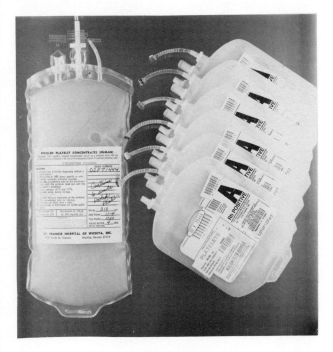

Pooled platelets.

Continued.

Table 7-1   Blood and blood components—cont'd

Product	Infusion Guidelines
Platelets (Random) *Volume* usual order 6 to 10 units *Filter* Special component filter; use of microaggregate filter may be controversial	slowly if danger of circulatory overload exists; maximum transfusion time: 4 hours *Comments:* ABO and Rh compatible preferred but not necessary; no cross match required; request blood bank to pool (combine units); required pooling time: 20 minutes; blood bank will not pool until ready to infuse product
Platelets (Apheresis) *Volume* 200 to 300 ml *Filter* Same as Platelets (Random)	Same as Platelets (Random) *Comments:* Arrangements must be made with blood center apheresis department before need; must be ABO and Rh compatible; cross match required unless red cell–free product is provided
Leukapheresis (Granulocytes) *Volume* 300 to 400 ml *Filter* Same as Platelets (Random)	Give *slowly* over 2-hour to 4-hour period; reactions are common—check vital signs every 15 minutes throughout transfusion; granulocytes should be transfused as soon as possible after collection but must be infused within 24 hours *Comments:* Same as Platelets (Apheresis) except red cell–free product; observe patient for a severe reaction indicated

Table 7-1   Blood and blood components—cont'd

Product	Infusion Guidelines
Leukapheresis (Granulocytes)	by cyanosis, shortness of breath, temperature above 104° F, and drop in blood pressure; febrile reactions occur in approximately two thirds of patients receiving leukocytes; the following laboratory work is usually ordered 1 hour after transfusion: WBC, differential, platelet count
Cryoprecipitate *Volume* 5 to 10 ml/unit; total of 10 ml normal saline is added in the blood bank; usual order 6 to 10 units *Filter* Special component filter	Rapid infusion: recommend 30 min to 1 hr *Comments:* Cross match not required; need not be ABO or Rh specific; each unit contains approximately 150 grams of fibrinogen and 80 units of Factor VIII; blood bank does not thaw and pool until requested; required preparation time: 20 minutes

Protocol for Blood and Blood Component Administration

Pretransfusion

1. Verify prescribed physician order for specific blood or blood component with the appropriate date of transfusion administration.
2. Obtain the patient's transfusion history, and report any incidence of previous adverse reaction during or after previous blood transfusion.
3. Follow agency-prescribed procedure for type and cross matching for blood and blood component therapy.
4. Establish patent peripheral or central line site. To ensure safety

of blood product administration for patients with multilumen catheters, reserve one lumen of the catheter for blood and blood component infusions. This technique minimizes the potential of infection for patients with these catheters.

5. Select appropriate tubing. All blood and components must be administered through a filter designed to retain blood clots and other debris. Follow agency policy for use of appropriate filter.

6. Blood bank personnel issuing the blood unit and nursing personnel administering the transfusion must identify the blood product, the identification number on the transfusion request, and the identical information on the recipient's medical record.

   a. The identification number and name on the patient's wrist band must be identical with the name and number on the transfusion unit and on the compatibility label.

   b. Donor's ABO and Rh group must be present on donor unit and transfusion request.

   c. Patient's (recipient) ABO and Rh group must be present on the transfusion request. Verify ABO and Rh compatibility between the patient (recipient) and donor.

   d. Check the expiration date on the blood bag.

   e. Inspect the blood product for any abnormalities.

   f. Ask the patient to identify himself by giving his complete name. If the patient is unable to state name, follow appropriate agency procedure in validating patient identification. *Never* administer blood to a patient without correct, appropriate, identifying bracelet or tag.

   g. Explain the procedure to the patient.

   h. Obtain written consent form if required by the agency.

   i. Inform the patient of potential adverse effects of blood transfusion (see Table 7-2) and instruct him to report symptoms experienced promptly to nurse or physician.

   j. Encourage the patient to ask questions about the procedure and potential adverse effects.

   k. On completion of the identification process, the person starting the transfusion and the other licensed person verifying the correct product must record date, time, and their signatures on the transfusion requisition.

Initiating the Transfusion

After following protocol to obtain the blood product from the blood bank, administer the blood product within 30 minutes, since blood can deteriorate and become rapidly contaminated at room temperature. (A blood product cannot be returned to the blood bank if the product is not initiated in appropriate time.)

The transfusion should be initiated slowly and then maintained at an administration rate appropriate for the patient's condition. All blood components should be infused within 4 hours; time the transfusion accurately.

During the first 15 minutes of initial transfusion, remain with the patient and protect him from adverse reactions. Note any adverse or unusual symptoms. The earlier these symptoms are detected, the more promptly the infusion can be discontinued and treatment instituted. (See Table 7-2 for effects and symptoms of blood transfusion.) Assess the patient on an ongoing basis. Take baseline vital signs (temperature, pulse, respirations, and blood pressure) before the transfusion and throughout the transfusion process.

Use only compatible IV fluids. Never inject any drug into a blood bag; only normal saline solution may be added to or run simultaneously with blood or components before or during transfusion.

Prevent damage to the blood cells. For infusing most blood components an 18-gauge catheter is appropriate. For patients with small veins (small children and the elderly), a thin-walled, 23-gauge ''scalp vein'' needle may be used. Also, consider use of a blood warmer for massive transfusions and transfusions in the neonate, child, or immunosuppressed patient.

Troubleshooting Tips

Sluggish IV lines and clogged filters that decrease the flow rate may be encountered during transfusion. Investigative questions to ask include:

- Is there a kink in the administration set?
- Is the correct gauge of needle or catheter being used?
- Has irrigation with normal saline been attempted?
- Has the filter been used for more than 2 units?
- Has the blood bag been rotated to distribute contents evenly?

- Is the blood bag 36 to 48 inches above the venipuncture site?
- Does the roller clamp need to be adjusted?

If all the above are negative or problems have been corrected, consider use of pressure cuff according to agency policy.

Posttransfusion

1. Complete posttransfusion documentation.
2. Return completed transfusion form to blood bank.
3. Continue to observe the patient, and monitor vital signs according to agency policy.
4. Dispose of used supplies in a puncture-proof, leakproof container; NOTE: if transfusion reaction occurs, return discontinued bag of blood and blood component with all attached solutions to the blood bank.
5. Follow up with prescribed, scheduled posttransfusion laboratory tests, for example, CBC, hemoglobin, hematocrit, platelet count, prothrombin time, or Factor VIII level.

Clinical Alert: Wear gloves while initiating and discontinuing a blood transfusion to protect from blood-borne infections (hepatitis, AIDS).

Adverse Effects of Blood Transfusion

Hemolytic (immediate and delayed) and febrile nonhemolytic reactions are the most frequent in occurrence of all the adverse effects listed. To provide immediate intervention for a transfusion reaction, the most common symptoms of a transfusion reaction and the appropriate interventions need to be studied. The greatest risk of exposure to infectious disease from blood transfusions is a 7% to 13% incidence of posttransfusion hepatitis. If the patient is suspected of having posttransfusion hepatitis, the blood bank service should be notified so that the donor can be investigated.

Table 7-2 lists in alphabetical order the most common adverse effects of blood transfusion and the potential symptoms the patient may experience.

Table 7-2   Adverse effects of blood transfusion

Reactions	Symptoms
Anaphylactic *Cause:* Previous sensitization by IgA-deficient patients who develop anti-IgA antibodies	Absence of fever, shock, respiratory distress, nausea, hypotension, abdominal cramps; occurs quickly following only a few milliliters of blood or plasma
Air Embolism *Cause:* Improper maintenance of a closed administration system	Shortness of breath, chest pain, cough, hypotension, cyanosis
Circulatory Overload *Cause:* Excessive or rapid volume of blood or blood component	Dyspnea, tightness in chest, dry cough, restlessness, severe headache, increased pulse and respiration
Citrate Toxicity *Cause:* Citrate anticoagulant accumulates, toxic effects due to ionized calcium in the blood, for example, hypocalcemia	Tingling in fingers, hypotension, nausea and vomiting, cardiac arrhythmias
Febrile Nonhemolytic *Cause:* Recipient anti-HLA antibodies react to transfused leukocyte or platelet antigens	Fever, flushing, chills, absent RBC hemolysis, lumbar pain, malaise, headache

Continued.

Table 7-2   Adverse effects of blood transfusion—cont'd

Reactions	Symptoms
Hemolytic *Immediate Cause:* Antibodies in recipient's plasma reacts to donor's antigens on red cells	Anxiety, increased pulse, respiration, and temperature, decreased blood pressure, dyspnea, nausea and vomiting, chills, hemoglobinemia, hemoglobinuria, abnormal bleeding, oliguria, shock; reactions may occur when as little as 10 to 15 ml of incompatible blood have been infused
Hemolytic *Delayed Cause:* Recipient becomes sensitized to foreign RBC antigens not in the ABO system	Occurs two or more days after transfusion; continued anemia, hemoglobinuria, lumbar pain
Hyperkalemia *Cause:* Prolonged storage of blood, releases potassium into the cell plasma	Onset within few minutes; EKG changes, peaked T-wave and widening of QRS, weakness of extremities, abdominal pain
Hypothemia *Cause:* Rapid administration of cold blood components	Shaking chills, hypotension, cardiac arrhythmias, cardiac arrest
Urticaria *Cause:* Allergy to a soluble product in the donor plasma	Local erythema, hives, and itching, usually without fever
Infections Transmitted by Transfusions	
Acquired Immune Deficiency Syndrome (AIDS) *Cause:* Donor blood HIV seropositive	Fever, night sweats, fatigue, weight loss, adenopathy, and skin lesions; seropositive for HIV virus

Table 7-2   Adverse effects of blood transfusion—cont'd

Reactions	Symptoms
Bacterial Contamination *Cause:* Contamination at time of donation or preparation; gram-negative bacteria release endotoxins	Onset within 2 hours of transfusion; chills, fever, abdominal pain, shock
Cytomegalovirus (CMV) CMV virus can exist in healthy adult	Immunosuppressed patients are at high risk (bone marrow transplant, open-heart surgery, newborn positive heterophil)—fatigue, weakness, adenopathy, low-grade fever
Hepatitis Hepatitis B more common than Hepatitis A	Occurs in a few weeks to months after transfusion; nausea and vomiting, jaundice, weakness, elevated liver enzyme levels
Graft-Versus-Host-Disease (GVHD) *Cause:* Immunocompetent donor; lymphocytes engraft and multiply in immunodeficient recipient	Bone marrow–suppressed patients at risk; fever, skin rash, diarrhea, presence of infection, jaundice
Malaria	Spiking fever after receiving transfusion containing red cells, platelets or fresh-frozen plasma; malaria organism isolated in the blood
Syphilis	Rare; blood test positive for syphilis
Thrombocytopenia Purpura	Occurs most often in women; decreased platelet count; generalized purplish rash

Management of Transfusion Reactions

The time between suspicion of a transfusion reaction and the initiation of appropriate therapy should be as short as possible. The nurse administering blood component therapy is responsible for obtaining baseline vital signs and monitoring the patient for any changes that may develop during and after any transfusion. An accurate assessment of clinical symptoms and reporting of this information is crucial in life-threatening reactions. Nursing staff should be skilled in blood component therapy, and policies and procedures for management of transfusion reactions should be readily available.

Guidelines established by the American Association of Blood Banks for blood transfusions include the following:

1. Stop the transfusion to limit the amount of blood infused.
2. Notify the physician.
3. Keep the IV line open with an infusion of normal saline.
4. Check all labels, forms, and patient identification to determine if the patient received the correct blood or component.
5. Report the suspected transfusion reaction to blood bank personnel immediately.
6. Send required blood samples, carefully drawn to avoid mechanical hemolysis, to the blood bank as soon as possible, together with the discontinued bag of blood, the administration set, attached IV solutions, and all the related forms and labels.
7. Send other samples, for example, urine for evaluation of acute hemolysis, as directed by the blood bank director or patient's physician.
8. Complete agency report of "Suspected Transfusion Reaction" form (if appropriate).
9. Medication and supplies to have nearby:
   a. Injectable: aminophylline, diphenhydramine hydrochloride (Benadryl), dopamine, epinephrine, heparin, hydrocortisone, furosemide (Lasix) Oral: acetaminophen, aspirin
   b. Oxygen setup, tubing, cannula, or mask, and airway device
   c. Foley catheterization kit
   d. Blood culture bottles

e. IV fluids (isotonic solution)

f. IV tubings

Clinical Alert: The nurse must become familiar with all the equipment used in the employing agency so that intervention for a transfusion reaction can be administered promptly and safely.

Documentation Recommendations

- Location of patent peripheral or central line IV site
- Baseline vital signs before transfusion
- Time transfusion was started
- Type of product and identification number
- Signature of person initiating the transfusion and signature of second licensed person verifying correct product
- Total number of units infused and their identification numbers
- Total volume of blood component and saline infused
- Time transfusion was completed
- Premedication or postmedication supplies (tubings) used for blood component therapy
- Patient's response to transfusion, especially any symptoms of an adverse reaction (chills, fever, urticaria, sweating, nausea, blood in urine, shortness of breath, dyspnea, hypotension, or anxiety)
- All nursing interventions initiated and performed in response to an adverse reaction

Nursing Diagnoses

- Fluid volume excess, potential, related to infusion of the product or volume of the infusion
- Infection, potential for, related to contamination of supplies or blood product
- Fluid volume deficit: actual or potential, related to loss of blood volume
- Cardiac output, altered: decreased

Patient/Family Teaching for Self-Management

- Describe purpose, schedule, and procedure for blood component administration.
- Explain the potential blood transfusion reactions (fever, chills,

urticaria, back pain, pain at infusion site, chest pain, dyspnea, and nausea) and the importance of reporting the reactions promptly to the nurse or physician.

■ Instruct the patient or caregiver regarding potential delayed reactions to transfusions, which may occur several hours, days, or a week after transfusion, for example, jaundice and generalized purplish rash (purpura); advise to notify the physician promptly.

■ If blood component therapy is to be administered in the home setting, assess availability of the caregiver to be present in the home during administration of the blood product.

Home Care Considerations

■ The patient must be *homebound* (unable to drive self or leave home without assistance).

■ The patient should be alert, cooperative, and able to respond appropriately to body symptoms.

■ The patient must have been previously transfused without difficulty.

■ A responsible adult must be present in the home to participate in the identification process and to summon assistance (physician or paramedic) if necessary.

■ Whole blood must not be administered in the home.

■ The blood specimen for type and cross match should be drawn 24 to 48 hours before blood product administration.

■ Each unit of the blood component therapy must be checked by a registered nurse and blood bank personnel before administration.

■ The registered nurse works under the directions of a physician in accordance with federal, state, and local regulations and the standards of the American Association of Blood Banks.

■ The registered nurse should be knowledgeable and skilled in the procedure of blood product administration.

■ The nurse must remain in attendance throughout the blood transfusion process and for at least 30 minutes after transfusion.

■ Blood is to be transported in insulated containers with ice packets that maintain the temperature between 1° and 10° C for 24 hours.

■ The container, empty bags, and tubing should be returned to the blood bank on completion of the transfusion.

- Posttransfusion instructions are given in writing, and the patient or caregiver is given the names and phone numbers of individuals available at all times to be called in the event of a delayed problem.
- The nurse will arrange for prescribed posttransfusion laboratory test to be completed, for example, red blood cells (hemoglobin, hematocrit), within 24 hours; platelets: 18 hours after transfusion.

Clinical Alert: Home care nursing personnel should be alert and prepared for possible transfusion reactions. The drugs and supplies necessary to manage these potential reactions must be readily available for use. Protocols for management of transfusion reactions should be clearly defined and easily accessible to home care nursing staff.

Pediatric Considerations

- Blood from the newborn is usually cross matched against the mother's serum, which contains equal or greater quantities of any antibodies present in the infant at birth.
- Dosage for children varies according to age and weight: calculate dosage in milliliters per kilogram of weight.
- Blood units are prepared in special units, for example, Pedipacks, which usually equal half a conventional adult unit.
- Red cell transfusions require strict infusion times, for example, calculate 5% of total product to be delivered and infuse this amount over the first 15 minutes; this method facilitates early detection of a potential hemolytic reaction.
- Use microaggregate filters in routine blood and blood component transfusions.
- The use of blood warmers prevents hypothermia leading to dysrhythmia.
- Use an electronic infusion pump to monitor and control accuracy in the drip rate.
- Use straight line IV tubing to minimize volume of saline infusion.
- Use the umbilical vein in the newborn as a means of venous access.
- Only qualified personnel (physicians and nurses) in an appropriate environment should perform exchange transfusion in the newborn, since this procedure requires advanced skills.

■ Explain the transfusion procedure to the parents, obtain their consent, and review the transfusion history of the child. Include the child in all the preparation, teaching, and procedure components for transfusion therapy

Chapter
Resources

Blood Product Administration Audit

	Yes	No	NA
1. Verify the physician order for specific product to be given on a stated date.			
2. Check appropriate laboratory data.			
3. Review transfusion history of the patient.			
4. Select correct tubing for the blood and blood product.			
5. Explain the procedure to the patient.			
6. Obtain baseline vital signs (BP, T, P, R).			
7. Identify the patient by name and by written ID number on the patient bracelet.			
8. Confirm blood unit number, ABO, Rh group, and expiration date of product on donor unit, patient transfusion request form, and patient identification number on patient bracelet with another licensed professional.			
9. Prime blood tubing, taking care to cover the entire filter.			
10. Initiate the transfusion slowly.			
11. Readjust the transfusion rate after 15 minutes to desired infusion rate.			
12. Use normal saline only for flushing of IV line.			
13. Take the patient's vital signs throughout the transfusion according to agency policy.			
14. Document the procedure according to agency policy.			
15. Return completed posttransfusion request to blood bank.			

Table 7-3   Risks and benefits of blood from various sources

Type	Community*	Autologous†	Parentologous‡	Directed§
Availability				
Time	Immediate	3 or more days	3 or more days	3 or more days
Quantity	Indefinite	3 to 4 units‖	2 to 6 units‖	Number recruited
Emergency use	Yes	No	No	No
Multiple components	Yes	No	No‖	No‖
HIV infection risk	1 to 5 years	None	Less than 1 to 5 years	1 to 5 years
Hepatitis risk¶	1% to 2%	None	1% to 2%	Greater than 1% to 2%
Compatibility	By test	Always	By test	By test
Antibody formation	Yes	No	Yes	Yes
Clerical error risk	Low	Low	Low	Low
Phlebotomy risk (Patient)	No	Yes	No	No
Emotional concern	Slight	Very low	Low	Low
Cost	Processing fee	Processing fee plus surcharge	Processing fee plus surcharge	Processing fee plus surcharge

*Community—donor is selected through community blood supply.
†Autologous—blood is previously banked by recipient and transfused at time of need, for example, elective major surgery.
‡Parentologous—blood donor is parent to child.
§Directed—blood donor is selected by recipient of transfusion, for example, compatible blood grouping family member.
‖With special arrangements, more units and possibly other components may be possible.
¶Estimated, based on the use of the two new surrogate tests.

PATIENT AND PROFESSIONAL INFORMATION BOOKLETS

The American Red Cross and the Public Health Service have available the following publications regarding the blood supply and AIDS:

- AIDS and the Blood Supply
- AIDS and the Health Care Workers
- AIDS and Your Job
- Caring for the AIDS Patient at Home
- AIDS and Your Children
- If Your Antibody Test is Positive
- AIDS, Sex and You

Chemotherapy Administration

8

Can cause cancer.

Chemotherapy is the use of cytotoxic drugs in the teatment of cancer. It is recognized as one of the four modalities—surgery, radiation therapy, chemotherapy, and immunotherapy—that provide cure, control, or palliation as a goal of therapy. Chemotherapy may be used separately or in conjunction with other modalities.

Nursing has major responsibilities in caring for patients who receive chemotherapeutic agents. It is important that nurses know treatment goals, drug classifications with modes of action, principles of tumor growth and cell kill, and administration protocol. Chemotherapeutic agents should be administered only by nurses who have been educated and are skilled in the various procedures. Patient and family education on the many aspects of chemotherapy (for example, procedure, potential side effects and toxicities, and follow-up care) requires competent nursing assessment and intervention. The nurse should encourage the patient and family to participate and become an integral part in planning and implementing care. These responsibilities offer many challenges for the nurse administering chemotherapy.

Principles of Chemotherapy

Cell Generation Cycle

Normal cells and cancer cells go through the same division cycle characterized by a sequential series of phases or steps (Figure 8-1). The length of time that it takes for a cell to complete the phase or cycle varies. This time is called generation time. Chemotherapeutic drugs are most active against frequently dividing cells. Normal cells with rapid growth changes most commonly affected by chemotherapeutic agents include bone marrow (platelets, red and white blood cells), hair follicles, mucosal lining of the gastrointestinal tract, skin, and germinal cells (sperm and ova).

156

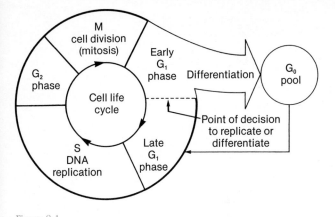

Figure 8-1
Cell generation cycle.
Courtesy Adria Laboratories, Columbus, Ohio.

Clinical Alert: Chemotherapy is given according to scheduled sequences or cycles that are planned to allow recovery of the normal cells. Anticipate expected changes, for example, low blood counts and hair loss, and incorporate these in the patient care plan.

Drug Classification

Chemotherapeutic agents are classified according to their pharmacologic action and their interference with cellular reproduction. The basic groups and their potential action are the following:

Cell cycle phase specific: Drugs that are active on cells undergoing division in the cell cycle.

G_1 Phase	G_2 Phase
Asparaginase	Bleomycin
Prednisone	Etoposide (VP-16)

S Phase	M Phase
Cytarabine (Ara-C)	Vinblastine

S Phase	M Phase
5-Fluorouracil	Vincristine
Hydroxyurea	Vindesine
Methotrexate	
6-Mercaptopurine	
6-Thioguanine	

Cell cycle phase nonspecific: Drugs that are active on cells in either a dividing or resting state.

Alkylating Agents	Nitrosureas
Busulfan (Myleran)	Carmustine (BCNU)
Chlorambucil (Leukeran)	Lomustine (CCNU)
Cisplatin	Semustine (MeCCNU)
Cyclophosphamide (Cytoxan)	Streptozocin (Zanosar)
Mechlorethamine (Nitrogen Mustard)	
Melphalan (Alkeran)	
Thiotepa	

Antibiotics	Miscellaneous
Dactinomycin	Dacarbazine
Daunorubicin	Procarbazine
Doxorubicin (Adriamycin)	
Mitomycin C	
Mithramycin	

The remaining group of drugs that affect tumor cell growth by altering the intracellular environment is hormone and steroid drugs. The mechanism of action for each drug is different and is not clearly defined.

Hormones	Corticosteroids
Androgens	Dexamethasone (Decadron)
Fluoxymesterone (Halotestin)	Hydrocortisone (Solu-Cortef)

Hormones	Corticosteroids
Testosterone	Prednisone
Progestins	Prednisolone
Megestrol acetate (Megace)	
Medroxyprogesterone acetate (Depro-Provera) (intramuscular)	
Medroxyprogesterone acetate (Provera) (oral)	

Estrogens	Antihormonal Agents
Diethylstilbestrol (DES)	Aminoglutethimide (Cytadren)
Conjugated estrogens (Premarin)	Flutamide Leuprolide
Chlorotrianisene (TACE)	Mitotane Tamoxifen

Clinical Alert: Become familiar with the potential side effects and toxicities associated with chemotherapeutic drugs in all categories.

Tumor Growth

The regulatory mechanism controlling the growth of cancer cells differs from that of normal cells. Unlike normal cells, cancer cells grow via a pyramid effect; however, they grow at the *same rate* as the tissue from which they originated. The time required for a tumor mass to reach a certain size is called doubling time. During early stages of tumor growth, doubling time is more rapid than later stages. This pattern of growth is called Gompertzian function (Figure 8-2).

Clinical Alert: Tumor cells are more sensitive to chemotherapeutic agents that are toxic to rapidly dividing cells. Treatment protocols for patients with leukemia and lymphoma may include interventions for rapid cell destruction. A protocol may include fluid hydration and administration of allopurinol to minimize renal toxicity 24 hours before the initial chemotherapeutic drug dose is given.

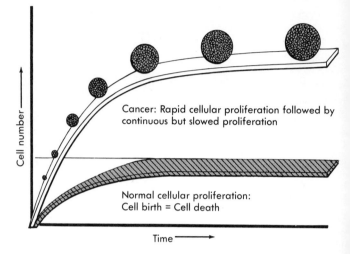

Figure 8-2
Gompertzian function.
From Goodman MS: Cancer: chemotherapy and care, Pt I, Bristol Laboratories,
Division of Bristol-Myers Co, Evansville, Ind.

Cell Kill Hypothesis

A single cancer cell is capable of multiplying and eventually killing
the host. The last tumor cell needs to be killed to achieve a cure in
the treatment of cancer. With each course of the drug therapy a
given dose of chemotherapeutic drug kills only a *fraction* and *not
all* of the cancer cells present. Repeated courses of chemotherapy
must then be used to reduce the total cancer cell number (Figure
8-3).

Clinical Alert: Repeated courses of chemotherapeutic drugs require anticipation of potential drug cumulative effects.

Factors Considered in Drug Selection

1. Patient's eligibility for chemotherapy (confirmed diagnosis,
   bone marrow, nutritional, hepatic, and renal status, expectation
   of longevity, previous history of chemotherapy and radiation
   therapy)
2. Cancer cell type (for example, squamous cell, adenocarcino-
   ma)

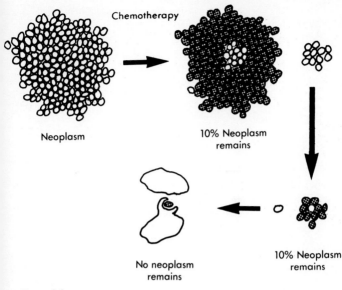

Figure 8-3
Cell kill hypothesis.
From Goodman MS: Cancer: chemotherapy and care, Pt I, Bristol Laboratories, Division of Bristol-Myers Co, Evansville, Ind.

3. Rate of drug absorption (for example, treatment interval and routes—oral, IV, intraperitoneal)
4. Tumor location (for example, many drugs do not cross the blood-brain barrier)
5. Tumor load (for example, larger tumors are generally less responsive to chemotherapy)
6. Tumor resistance to chemotherapy (for example, tumor cells can mutate and produce variant cells distinct from the tumor stem cell of origin)

Combination Chemotherapy

Chemotherapeutic drugs are most frequently given in combination. This process enhances the effect of the drugs on the tumor cell kill. Considerations for drugs used in combination include effectiveness as a single agent, results in increased tumor cell kill, increased patient survival, presence of a synergistic action, varied toxicities, different mechanisms of action, and administration in repeated courses to minimize the immunosuppressive effects that might otherwise occur. An example of combination chemotherapy is the widely known MOPP regimen—Nitrogen *M*ustard, vincristine (*O*ncovin), *p*rocarbazine, and *p*rednisone—used in treatment for patients with Hodgkin's disease.

Chemotherapy Administration

Drug Dosage Calculation

Drug dosage for cancer chemotherapy is based on BSA in both adults and children. Drug calculations should be verified by a second person to ensure dose accuracy. The dosage range of one drug may vary with different drug regimens. (See Chapter 4 for specifics of drug calculations.)

Drug Reconstitution

Prepare and reconstitute drugs using aseptic technique in accordance with current manufacturer's recommendations. Label all syringes of reconstituted drugs immediately with the name of the drug. Many of the chemotherapeutic agents are colorless and cannot be distinguished from each other after reconstitution. (See "Safe Handling Recommendations for Drug Preparation Guidelines.")

Route of Administration Guidelines

  I. *Oral*—emphasize importance of patient compliance to follow prescribed schedule.
 II. *Subcutaneous and intramuscular*—may require demonstration with a return demonstration if the patient is receiving prescribed self-injections. Be sure to rotate injection sites for each dose.
III. *Topical*—cover surface area with thin film of medication; instruct the patient to wear loose-fitting, cotton clothing. Wear gloves and be sure to wash hands thoroughly after procedure. Caution the patient not to touch area of topical ointment application.
 IV. *Intraarterial*—requires catheter placement in artery near tumor site; because of arterial pressure administer the drug by means of an infusion pump. Instruct the patient and family

on care components of catheter and infusion pumps if chemotherapy is given in home setting.

V. *Intracavity*—instill the drug into the bladder through a catheter and/or through a chest tube into the pleural cavity. Follow prescribed premedication dosage to minimize potential local irritation caused by drugs given through the intracavity route.

VI. *Intraperitoneal*—deliver the drug into the abdominal cavity through the implantable port and/or external suprapubic catheter. Monitor the patient for abdominal pressure, pain, and fever (Figure 8-4).

VII. *Intrathecal*—reconstitute all intrathecal medications with preservative-free, sterile normal saline or sterile water. Infusion of medication may be given through an Ommaya reservoir, if available, and/or through lumbar puncture procedure. Usual volume of medication instilled is 15 ml or less (Figure 8-5).

VIII. *IV*—may be given through central venous catheters or peripheral venous access. Methods of IV administration include the following:

    A. *Push:* (bolus)—medication is administered through syringe by direct IV method.

    B. *Piggyback:* (secondary setup)—drug is administered using a secondary bag (bottle) and tubing; primary infusion

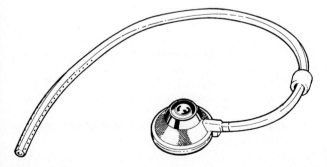

Figure 8-4
Implantable intraperitoneal port.
Courtesy CR Bard, Inc, Cranston, RI.

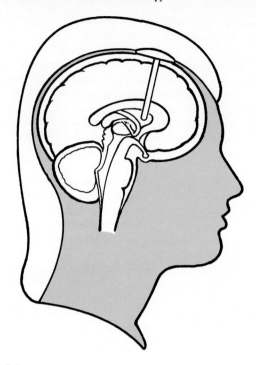

Figure 8-5
The Ommaya reservoir.
From Brager B and Yasko J: Care of the client receiving chemotherapy, Reston, Va., 1984, Reston Publishing Co, Inc.

is concurrently maintained throughout drug administration.

C. *Side arm:* drug is administered through syringe and needle into side port of a running (free-flowing) IV infusion.

D. *Infusion:* drug is added to prescribed volume of fluid IV bag (bottle).

Clinical Alert: Check for blood return before, during, and after infusion of chemotherapeutic drugs. Follow the agency guidelines for frequency of monitoring continuous chemotherapeutic infusions. For vesicant drug continuous infusion, suggestions include validating blood return every two hours; for nonvesicant drug continuous infusion, validate blood return every four hours.

Vein Selection and Venipuncture

Many chemotherapeutic agents can be irritating to veins and surrounding tissues. Peripheral sites should be changed daily before administration of vesicants. (See "Management of Extravasation.") The number of available veins may be limited as a result of previous therapy. (See Chapter 2.)

Procedure for Chemotherapeutic Drug Administration

1. Verify patient identification, drug, dose, route, and time of administration with the physician's order.
2. Review drug allergy history with the patient.
3. Review appropriate laboratory data and other tests.
4. Verify informed consent for treatment.
5. Select appropriate equipment and supplies.
6. Calculate the dose and reconstitute the drug using aseptic technique (follow safe handling guidelines).
7. Explain the procedure to patient and family. (See "Patient Teaching.")
8. Administer prescribed antiemetics or other medications.
9. Initiate peripheral IV site or prepare central venous access site.
10. Administer chemotherapeutic agents.
11. Monitor patient at scheduled frequencies throughout course of drug administration.
12. Anticipate and plan interventions for potential side effects or major system toxicity. (See Tables 8-1 and 8-2.)
13. Dispose of all used supplies and unused drugs into approved puncture-proof, leakproof containers outside of patient area.
14. Document procedure according to agency policy and procedure. (See "Documentation Recommendations.")

Chemotherapeutic Toxicities

Chemotherapeutic drugs have the potential for causing adverse side effects and major system toxicity and dysfunction in patients receiving these agents. Each side effect and toxicity varies in severity according to the patient's individual response to the drug therapy. Nursing responsibilities include evaluating individual patient response to the drugs, teaching the patient or caregiver self-management interventions, and monitoring various laboratory data and symptoms observed or reported by the patient.

The information listed in Tables 8-1 and 8-2 may be referred to in developing the plan of care for the patient receiving chemotherapeutic drugs.   *Text continued on p. 178.*

Table 8-1   Patient teaching for self-management of most common side effects from chemotherapeutic drugs

Side Effects	Points to Cover
Aches and Pains *Nursing action:* Assess location, quality, and duration of pain	Pain medication should be taken on a regular schedule Side effects of pain medicine are constipation, dry mouth, and drowsiness Rest and relaxation strategies include music, progressive relaxation exercise, distraction, and positive imaging
Alopecia *Hair loss* Adriamycin, cyclophosphamide (Cytoxan), daunorubicin (DTIC), vinblastine *Hair thinning* 5-FU, methotrexate, bleomycin, vincristine, etoposide (VP-16) *Nursing action:* Discourage use of scalp tourniquets for patients with diseases that originate with or metastasize to the scalp	Hair loss occurs 10 to 21 days after drug treatment Hair loss is temporary, and hair will regrow when drug is stopped Hair loss may occur suddenly and in large amounts Select wig, cap, scarf, or turban before hair loss occurs Avoid use of hair dryers, curling irons, and harsh or frequent shampoos

Table 8-1   Patient teaching for self-management of most
common side effects from chemotherapeutic drugs—cont'd

Side Effects	Points to Cover
Anorexia	Eating is a social event; eat with others in a pleasant area with soft music and attractive settings
	Freshen up before meals, for example, mouth care, exercise
	Small, frequent meals (five to six meals daily)
	Avoid drinking fluids with meals to prevent feeling of fullness
	Concentrate on eating foods high in protein, for example, eggs, milk products, peanut butter, tuna, beans, peas
	Breakfast may be the most tolerable meal of the day; try to include one third of daily calories at this time
	Monitor and record weight weekly; report weight loss
Constipation Drugs associated with potential: vincristine, vinblastine, and narcotics *Nursing action:* Determine normal bowel habits; advise the patient not to strain with bowel evacuation	Increase intake of high-fiber foods, for example, whole grain products, bran, fresh fruit, raw vegetables, popcorn
	Increase fluid intake to 2 to 3 quarts of liquids daily; encourage fresh fruit juices, prunes, and/or hot liquids on waking
	Follow prescribed scheduled use of stool softener
	Follow prescribed physician orders if no bowel movement for 3 days or more

Continued.

Table 8-1   Patient teaching for self-management of most common side effects from chemotherapeutic drugs—cont'd

Side Effects	Points to Cover
Cystitis Drug associated with potential: cyclophosphamide *Nursing action:* Observe urine for color and amount, and assess frequency of voiding; advise patient to take oral cyclophosphamide (Cytoxan) early in the day	Increase fluid intake to 3 quarts daily Empty bladder at least every 4 hours, especially at bedtime and at least once during the night Report increasing symptoms of frequency, bleeding, and temperature elevations promptly to the physician
Diarrhea *Nursing action:* Monitor serum fluid and electrolytes	Avoid eating high-roughage, greasy, and spicy foods; avoid using milk products or use boiled skim milk Eat a bland diet Increase fluid intake to 3 quarts of liquids daily (weak, tepid tea, bouillon, grape juice) Record number and consistency of daily bowel movements; report information to the physician Follow prescribed medication schedule if problem persists beyond 1 day Cleanse rectal area after each bowel movement
Depression *Nursing action:* Assess for changes in mood, affect	Set small goals that are achievable daily Participate in enjoyable and diversionary activities, for example, music, reading, outings Share feelings and concerns with someone

Table 8-1 Patient teaching for self-management of most common side effects from chemotherapeutic drugs—cont'd

Side Effects	Points to Cover
Fatigue *Nursing action:* Assess for possible causes (anemia, chronic pain, stress, depression, and insufficient rest or nutritional intake)	Conserve energy; rest when tired Plan for gradual accommodation of activities into life-style Monitor dietary and fluid intake daily
Hematopoietic Changes *Leukopenia* Most myelosuppressive agents produce WBC nadir 7 to 14 days after drug administration *Nursing action:* Monitor white blood count and differential; change equipment as indicated, for example, O_2 set up, IV supplies; teach sexual hygiene	Avoid sources of infection, for example, people with bacterial infections, colds, sore throats, flu, chicken pox, measles, and cold sores Avoid having fresh fruit, plants, and flowers at or near bedside Avoid cleaning animal litter boxes Maintain good personal hygiene, for example, bathe daily, wash hands before eating and preparing food, clean carefully after bowel movements, keep nails clean and clipped short and straight across Maintain adequate fluid intake Conserve energy; get adequate rest and exercise Prevent trauma to skin and mucous membranes Avoid elective dental work or surgery Avoid enemas, rectal suppositories and temperatures, and catheterizations

Continued.

Table 8-1   Patient teaching for self-management of most
common side effects from chemotherapeutic drugs—cont'd

Side Effects	Points to Cover
Hematopoietic Changes *Leukopenia*	Use toothettes or nonabrasive dental cleaning devices Report signs and symptoms of infection immediately to the physician; for example, fever of 38° C or greater, cough, sore throat, a shaking chill, and painful or frequent urination
Thrombocytopenia Drugs associated with a delayed cumulative effect: mitomycin, and nitrosureas *Nursing action:* Monitor platelet counts; observe bleeding precautions; apply firm pressure to venipuncture site for 3 to 5 minutes; monitor pad count on menstruating females; monitor environment for sharp objects	Avoid use of straight-edge razor, power tools, physical activity causing injury Avoid use of drugs containing aspirin Humidify the air; use lotion and lubricants on skin and lips Avoid invasive procedures; no intramuscular injections Discourage bare feet when ambulatory Use sanitary pads instead of tampons Report the following signs and symptoms immediately to the physician: bleeding gums, increased bruising, petechiae, purpura, hypermenorrhea, tarry-colored stools, blood in urine, or coffee-ground emesis

Table 8-1 Patient teaching for self-management of most
common side effects from chemotherapeutic drugs—cont'd

Side Effects	Points to Cover
Hematopoietic Changes *Anemia* *Nursing action:* Monitor hematocrit and hemoglobin, especially during drug nadir	Adjust physical activity to accommodate periods of rest Report the following signs and symptoms promptly to the physician, fatigue, dizziness, shortness of breath, and palpitations
Nausea and Vomiting *Nursing action:* Premedicate with antiemetic before nausea begins, for example, one-half hour before meals; patient may require routine antiemetics for 3 to 5 days following some chemotherapy protocols; monitor fluid and electrolyte status	Eat frequent, small meals Avoid greasy or fatty foods and very sweet foods or candies Avoid unpleasant sights, odors and tastes Cold foods, salty foods, dry crackers, and dry toast may be more tolerable If vomiting is severe, restrict diet to clear liquids and notify the physician Consider diversionary activities, for example, music therapy and relaxation techniques Report weight loss to physician
Mucositis, Rectal *Nursing action:* Monitor for electrolyte imbalance and granulocyte count; monitor number, consistency and amount of bowel movements and urine output; assess for rectal bleeding	Eat low-residue and easily digestible foods Increase intake of liquids to replace fluid loss Follow prescribed medication schedule, for example, antidiarrheal and pain control drugs

Continued.

Table 8-1   Patient teaching for self-management of most common side effects from chemotherapeutic drugs—cont'd

Side Effects	Points to Cover
Mucositis, Vaginal Symptoms occur 3 to 5 days after chemotherapy and subside in 7 to 10 days after therapy	Report pain, ulceration, or bleeding of mucous membranes lining the perineum and vagina to physician Sitz bath with warm salt water may provide relief of vaginal itching and odor Use hydrogen peroxide (one-quarter strength) with warm water after voiding to rinse perineal area Avoid commercial douches
Pharyngitis and Esophagitis	Eat a soft pureed or liquid diet Follow prescribed scheduled medication to relieve discomfort Report to the physician symptoms that persist more than 3 days
Skin Changes	Maintain good personal hygiene Use topical preparations to minimize itching Avoid use of perfume and perfumed lotion Avoid scratching to prevent infection
Stomatitis (Oral) Symptoms occur 5 to 7 days after chemotherapy and persist up to 10 days	Continue brushing regularly; use soft toothbrush Use non-irritant mouthwash, for example, salt, soda and water solution, at least four times daily Avoid irritants to the mouth, for example, tobacco, al-

Table 8-1 Patient teaching for self-management of most common side effects from chemotherapeutic drugs—cont'd

Side Effects	Points to Cover
Stomatitis (Oral)	coholic beverages, spices, and commercial mouth-washes
	Avoid wearing dentures until mouth soreness heals
	Maintain good nutritional intake; eat soft or liquid foods high in protein; add sauces or gravies in food to make food soupier
	Follow prescribed medication schedule, for example, drugs for oral candidiasis
	Report promptly to physician persistent symptoms, and if white patches occur on tongue, back of throat, or gums

Table 8-2 Major system toxicity or dysfunction and nursing management

Toxicity/Dysfunction	Nursing Management
Cardiac Toxicity	Verify baseline cardiac studies, for example, EKG, ejection fracture; cardiac enzymes, before drug administration
Drugs associated with potential: doxorubicin and daunorubicin	Monitor cardiac status and report symptoms regarding tachycardia, shortness of breath, distended neck veins, gallop heart rhythm, and ankle edema

Continued.

Table 8-2   Major system toxicity or dysfunction and nursing
management—cont'd

Toxicity/Dysfunction	Nursing Management
Cardiac Toxicity	Monitor and record total cumulative dose of drug in the patient's medical record; adriamycin approximate maximum lifetime dose is 550 mg/m^2
Hematopoietic Toxicity (See Table 8-1)	
Hepatic Toxicity Drugs associated with potential: adriamycin, asparaginase, BCNU, CCNU, methotrexate, mercaptopurine, mithramycin, and streptozocin	Monitor liver function studies, for example, lactic dehydrogenase (LDH), bilirubin, prothrombin time, and liver function tests—serum glutamic-oxaloacetic transaminase (SGOT) and serum glutamic-pyruvic transaminase (SGPT) Report to the physician signs of jaundice, tenderness over the liver, and urine and stool color changes
Hypersensitivity Reaction Drugs associated with potential: asparaginase, doxorubicin (local erythema), and bleomycin	Review the patient's allergy history Monitor for symptoms of hypersensitivity and anaphylaxis, for example, agitation, urticaria, rash, chills, cyanosis, bronchospasm, abdominal cramping, and hypotension; onset may be rapid or delayed; advise the patient to report subjective symptoms promptly Ensure proper medical equipment is nearby and

Table 8-2 Major system toxicity or dysfunction and nursing management—cont'd

Toxicity/Dysfunction	Nursing Management
Hypersensitivity Reaction	in good working condition Emergency drugs for intervention should be readily available When administering a drug with potential for a reaction, give a test dose, monitor vital signs, and observe for allergic response If allergic response occurs, stop drug administration and notify the physician immediately
Metabolic Alterations	
Hypocalcemia	Monitor serum level; observe for symptoms of muscle cramping, tingling of extremities, depression, and tetany
Hypercalcemia	Monitor serum level; observe for anorexia, constipation, nausea, vomiting, polyuria, and mental status change
Hypoglycemia	Monitor serum and urine levels; observe for symptoms of weakness, diaphoresis, hunger, headache, and tachycardia
Hyperglycemia	Monitor serum and urine levels; observe for symptoms of thirst, hunger, glucosuria, and weight loss

Continued.

Table 8-2 Major system toxicity or dysfunction and nursing management—cont'd

Toxicity/Dysfunction	Nursing Management
Hyperuricemia Potential with treatment of highly proliferative tumors, for example, leukemia and lymphoma	Monitor serum and urine levels; daily intake and output Initiate prescribed drug therapy (for example, allopurinol) to inhibit the formation of uric acid before administration of chemotherapy drug Provide vigorous hydration, for example, oral and IV fluid intake (2000 to 3000 ml), beginning 12 to 24 hours before initiation of chemotherapy Report symptoms of pain, chills, fever, and diminished urinary output
Hypokalemia	Monitor serum level; observe for symptoms of muscle weakness, and twitches, paralytic ileus, and polyuria
Hyperkalemia	Monitor serum level; observe for symptoms of confusion, complaints of numbness or tingling, weakness, and cardiac arrhythmias
Hypomagnesemia	Monitor serum level; observe for symptoms of personality changes, anorexia, nausea, vomiting, lethargy, weakness, and tetany

Table 8-2 Major system toxicity or dysfunction and nursing management—cont'd

Toxicity/Dysfunction	Nursing Management
Neurotoxicity Drugs associated with potential: vincristine, vinblastine, intrathecal cytarabine, methotrexate infusions, high peak plasma levels of 5-FU, and high doses of ARA-C and cisplatin	Monitor and report symptoms of weakness, numbness, and tingling sensation of hands, arms, and feet; also monitor and report symptoms of hoarseness, jaw pain, hallucinations, mental depression, decreased or absent deep tendon reflexes, slapping gait or foot drop, severe constipation, and paralytic ileus
Ototoxicity Drug associated with potential: cisplatin	Verify baseline audiogram Monitor and report symptoms of tinnitus, hearing loss, and vertigo
Pulmonary Toxicity Drugs associated with potential: bleomycin, busulfan, carmustine	Verify baseline respiratory function Individuals older than age 70 years have increased risk Monitor respiratory status and report symptoms of dyspnea, dry cough, rales, tachypnea, and fever
Reproductive System Dysfunction Drugs associated with potential: chlorambucil, cyclophosphamide, mechlorethamine	Assess for nature and frequency of sexual dysfunction Counsel with the patients regarding avoidance of pregnancy and sperm banking before chemotherapy administration; provide information on contraceptives

Continued.

Table 8-2   Major system toxicity or dysfunction and nursing management—cont'd

Toxicity/Dysfunction	Nursing Management
Reproduction System Dysfunction	Inform the patients of potential for temporary or permanent infertility and loss of libido
	Women may experience symptoms including amenorrhea, "hot flashes," insomnia, dyspareunia, and vaginal dryness; estrogen therapy may be helpful in management of these symptoms
Renal System Toxicity	Verify baseline renal function
Drugs associated with potential: cisplatin, cyclophosphamide, methotrexate, mithramycin, and streptozotocin	Encourage adequate fluid intake
	Monitor intake and output, weight changes
	Report diminished output to physician, for example, less than 500 ml in 24 hours

Safe Handling of Chemotherapeutic Agents

The number and usage of chemotherapeutic agents have increased considerably in recent years. A concern among health care workers has emerged regarding the potential occupational hazard associated with the handling of these drugs. Clinical studies have indicated that many agents are carcinogenic, mutagenic, and teratogenic or any combination of the three. The exposure to these chemotherapeutic agents can occur from inhalation, absorption, and digestion. Recommended safe handling practice guidelines should be referred to when implementing policy and procedure practices within each agency that prepares, administers, stores, or disposes of supplies or unused chemotherapeutic agents.*

Safe handling practice guidelines include the following:

- Drug preparation
- Drug administration
- Disposal of supplies and unused drugs
- Management of chemotherapy spill
- Caring for patients receiving chemotherapy, for example, linen contamination, patient excreta
- Staff education
- Employment practice regarding reproductive issues

Drug Preparation

To ensure safe handling, all chemotherapeutic drugs should be prepared according to the package insert in a class II biological safety cabinet (BSC). Venting to the outside is preferable where feasible. Personal protective equipment includes disposable surgical latex gloves and a gown made of lint-free, low-permeability fabric with a closed front, long sleeves, and elastic or knit cuffs. Wear eye-protective splash goggles or face shield when preparing drugs if not using a biological safety cabinet.

Suggestions to minimize exposure:

- Wash hands before and after drug handling
- Limit access to drug preparation area
- Keep labeled drug spill kit near preparation area
- Apply gloves before drug handling
- Prepare drugs using aseptic technique
- Avoid eating, drinking, smoking, chewing gum, applying cosmetics, or storing food in or near drug preparation area
- Place absorbent pad on work surface
- Use Luer-Lok equipment
- Open drug vials or ampules away from body
- Vent vials with a hydrophobic filter needle or pin to prevent spray of drug
- Wrap alcohol wipe around neck of ampule before opening
- Prime lines containing drugs inside BSC using original drug vial or a zip-lock bag

---

*Recommendations for safe handling of chemotherapeutic drugs are available from the Occupational Safety and Health Administration (OSHA), National Cytotoxic Study Commission, and American Society of Hospital Pharmacists.

- Cover tip of needle with sterile gauze or alcohol wipe when expelling air from syringe
- Label all chemotherapeutic drugs
- Clean up any spills immediately
- Transport drugs to delivery area in a leakproof container

Clinical Alert: Change gloves between drug preparation and administration and at least every 30 minutes during drug preparation or administration to ensure maximum protection.

Drug Administration

1. Wear protective equipment (gloves, gown, and eyewear) as mentioned in ''Drug Preparation.''
2. Inform the patient that chemotherapeutic drugs are harmful to normal cells and that protective measures used by personnel minimize their exposure to these drugs throughout their workday.
3. Administer drugs in a safe and unhurried environment.
4. Place a plastic-backed absorbent pad under the tubing during administration to catch any leakage.
5. Do not dispose of any supplies or unused drugs in patient care areas. (See ''Disposal of Supplies.'')

Disposal of Supplies and Unused Drugs

1. Avoid clipping or recapping needles and breaking syringes.
2. Place all supplies used *intact* in a leakproof, puncture-proof, appropriately labeled container.
3. Place all unused drugs in containers into a leakproof, puncture-proof, appropriately labeled container; position these containers in every area where drugs are prepared or administered so that waste materials need not be moved from one area to another.
4. Disposal of containers filled with chemotherapeutic supplies and unused drugs should be in accordance with regulations regarding hazardous wastes, for example, licensed sanitary landfill or incineration at 1000° C.

Management of Chemotherapy Spills

Chemotherapy spills should be cleaned up immediately by properly protected personnel trained in the appropriate procedures. A spill should be identified with a warning sign so that other persons in the area will not be contaminated. Recommended supplies and procedures to manage a chemotherapy spill on hard surfaces, linens, personnel, or patients include:

I. Supplies
   A. Chemotherapy spill kit:
      1. Respirator mask for airborne powder spills
      2. Plastic safety glasses or goggles
      3. Heavy-duty rubber gloves
      4. Absorbent pads to contain liquid spills
      5. Absorbent towels for clean-up after spill
      6. Small scoop to collect glass fragments
      7. Two large waste disposal bags
   B. Protective disposable gown (see ''Drug Preparation'')
   C. Containers of detergent solution and clear tap water for postspill cleanup
   D. Approved chemotherapy waste disposal puncture-proof and leakproof container
   E. Approved, specially labelled, impervious laundry bag
   F. Eye wash faucet adapters or fountain available in or near work area

II. Procedure for spill on hard surface
   A. Restrict area of spill.
   B. Obtain drug spill kit.
   C. Put on protective gown, gloves, and goggles (respirator mask if powder spill).
   D. Open waste disposal bags (double bag).
   E. Place absorbent pads gently on the spill; be careful not to touch spill.
   F. Place saturated absorbent pad into waste bag.
   G. Cleanse surface with absorbent towels using detergent solution and then wipe clean with clean tap water.
   H. Place all contaminated materials, for example, gown, gloves, saturated absorbent pads, and towels into double-bagged waste disposal bags.
   I. Discard waste bag with contents into approved waste disposal container.
   J. Wash hands thoroughly with soap and water.

III. Procedure for spill on linen
   A. Restrict area of spill.

B. Obtain drug spill kit.

C. Obtain specially marked, approved laundry bag and a labelled, impervious bag.

D. Put on protective gown, gloves, goggles.

E. Remove soiled, contaminated linen from the patient's bedside.

F. Place linen in approved, specially marked, impervious laundry bag.

G. Contaminated linen should be washed two times in laundry; laundry personnel should wear surgical latex gloves and gown when handling this material.

H. Clean contaminated area with absorbent towels and detergent solution.

I. Place all contaminated supplies used for management of spill into waste disposal bag and discard into approved waste disposal container.

J. Wash hands thoroughly with soap and water.

IV. Procedure for spill on personnel or patient

A. Restrict area of spill.

B. Obtain drug spill kit.

C. Immediately remove contaminated protective garments or linen.

D. Wash affected skin area with soap and water.

E. Eye exposure; immediately flood the affected eye with water for at least 5 minutes; obtain medical attention promptly.

F. Properly care for contaminated linen. (See ''Procedure for Spill on Linen.'')

G. Notify the physician if drug spills on patient.

V. Documentation

A. Document in the patient's medical record management of drug spill and notification of the patient's physician.

B. Document on the agency's approved forms management of spill occurring on hard surface, linen, or personnel.

Caring for Patients Receiving Chemotherapeutic Drugs

Personnel handling blood, vomitus, or excreta from patients who have received chemotherapy within the previous 48 hours should wear disposable surgical latex gloves and gowns to be discarded after use. (See ''Disposal of Supplies.'') Linen contaminated with chemotherapeutic drugs, blood, vomitus, or excreta from a patient who has received these drugs up to 48 hours before should be placed in a specially marked, impervious laundry bag. (See "Drug Spill on Linen.")

Staff Education

All personnel involved in any aspect of the handling of chemotherapeutic agents should receive an orientation to chemotherapy drugs, including their known risks, relevant techniques and procedures for handling, the proper use of protective equipment and materials, spill procedures, and medical policies; personnel handling chemotherapeutic agents includes those who are pregnant or actively trying to conceive children (per OSHA requirements). Evaluation of staff compliance may be achieved by quality monitoring on a regular basis. (See "Chapter Resources" for an example of audit tool.)

Employment Practices Regarding Reproductive Issues

The handling of chemotherapeutic agents by women who are either pregnant or actively trying to conceive, and by those who are breast-feeding remains a sensitive and unsettled issue. Suggestions have been made to offer these personnel the opportunity to transfer to areas that do not involve chemotherapeutic agents. All safe handling guidelines should be practiced with utmost care by all pregnant personnel.

Extravasation Management

Definition

Extravasation is the accidental infiltration of vesicant chemotherapeutic drugs from the vein into surrounding tissues at the IV site. Injuries that may occur as the result of extravasation include sloughing of tissue, infection, pain, and loss of mobility of an extremity. The degree of tissue damage is related to several factors such as drug concentration, the quantity of drug extravasated, and individual tissue responses.

Clinical Studies

Because of the harmful effect of vesicants on tissues, studies using patients as subjects are ethically and morally prohibitive. As a result, controlled clinical trials demonstrating effectiveness of treatment have been difficult to attain. Most extravasation interventions have been based on preclinical studies using animal model systems including mice, pigs, rabbits, and dogs. Treatment strategies for extravasation management include the use of specific antidotes based on their mechanism of action and guidelines for immediate intervention to minimize the tissue damage. Prevention of the extravasation and prompt intervention are the key elements for successful extravasation management.

Controversial Issues*

The management of extravasation of chemotherapeutic drugs involves some controversial issues. These issues include:

I. Use of antecubital fossa for drug administration
   A. Favoring antecubital fossa access
      1. Larger veins permit more rapid infusion of drug.
      2. Larger veins permit potentially irritating drugs to reach the general circulation sooner with less irritation.
   B. Opposing antecubital fossa access
      1. Arm mobility is restricted.
      2. Infiltration could cause extensive reconstructive efforts.
      3. Early infiltration may be difficult to assess.
      4. Potential for venous fibrosis; blood drawing from antecubital fossa may be more difficult.

II. Methods of drug sequencing
   A. Favoring the administration of vesicants first
      1. Vascular integrity decreases over time.
      2. Initial assessment of vein patency is most accurate.
      3. There is a potential for diminishing patient awareness of symptoms related to drug infiltration.
   B. Favoring the administration of vesicants last
      1. Vesicants are irritating and may increase vein fragility.
      2. Venous spasm may occur at onset of drug administration and alter assessment of venous access.

III. Needle or catheter size
   A. Favoring the use of larger gauge, for example 18- or 19-gauge

*Adapted from Oncology Nursing Society Task Force: Cancer chemotherapy guidelines and recommendations for nursing education and practice, 1988 guidelines, Pittsburgh, 1988, The Society.

1. Potential irritating chemotherapeutic agents can reach circulation sooner with less irritating effect on the peripheral veins.

B. Favoring the use of smaller gauge, for example, 20- or 23-gauge

1. Smaller-gauge devices are less likely to puncture the wall of a small vein.
2. Increased blood flow around a smaller-gauge device increases dilution of chemotherapeutic agents.
3. Phlebitis may be minimized with a smaller-gauge device.

Prevention of Extravasation

Nursing staff responsibilities for the prevention of extravasation include:

- Knowledge of drugs with vesicant potential (see Table 8-4)
- Skill in drug administration
- Identification of risk factors, for example, multiple venipunctures, previous treatment
- Anticipation of extravasation and knowledge of approved management protocol
- Obtaining a new venipuncture site daily if peripheral access used
- Consideration of central venous access for difficult peripheral access
- Administration of drug given in a quiet, unhurried environment
- Testing vein patency without using chemotherapeutic agents
- Providing adequate drug dilution, for example, side port infusion via free-flowing IV infusion
- Careful observation (visualize access site, extremity) throughout the procedure
- Validation of blood return from IV site before, during, and after vesicant drug infusion
- Educating patients regarding symptoms of drug infiltration, for example, pain, burning, and stinging sensations at IV site

Table 8-3.   Chemotherapeutic drugs, nonvesicants

Generic Name	Trade Name
Asparaginase	Elspar
Bleomycin	Blenoxane
Cisplatinum	Cisplatin
Cyclophosphamide	Cytoxan
Cytarabine	ARA-C, Cytosar
Floxuridine	FUDR
Fluorouracil	5-FU
Methotrexate	Mexate
Mitoxantrone	Novantrone
Thiophosphoramide	Thiotepa

Table 8-4.   Chemotherapeutic drugs with vesicant potential

Generic Name	Trade Name
Dacarbazine	DTIC-Dome
Dactinomycin	Actinomycin D, Cosmegen
Daunorubicin	Cerubidine, Daunomycin
Doxorubicin	Adriamycin
Mechlorethamine	Nitrogen Mustard, Mustargen
Mitomycin	Mutamycin
Plicamycin	Mithracin
Streptozocin	Zanosar
Vinblastine	Velban
Vincristine	Oncovin
Vindesine	Eldisine

Table 8-5.   Chemotherapeutic drugs with irritant potential

Generic Name	Trade Name
Carmustine	BCNU
Etoposide	VP-16, VePesid
Mitoguazone	Methyl-GAG, MGBG
Teniposide	VM-26

Protocol for Extravasation Management (Peripheral Site)

Agency policy and procedure for management of extravasation with the responsible physician's prescription should be easily accessible to the staff. The approved antidotes should be readily available, and the following procedure should be initiated with a physician's prescription as soon as extravasation of a vesicant or irritant agent is suspected or occurs.

1. Stop the administration of the chemotherapeutic drug.
2. Leave the needle or catheter in place.
3. Aspirate any residual drug and blood in the IV tubing, needle or catheter, and suspected infiltration site.
4. Instill the IV antidote (see Table 8-6).
5. Remove the needle.
6. If unable to aspirate the residual drug from the IV tubing, remove needle or catheter.
7. Inject the antidote subcutaneously clockwise into the infiltrated site using 25-gauge needle; change the needle with each new injection.
8. Avoid applying pressure to the suspected infiltration site.
9. Photograph the suspected area of extravasation according to agency's policy and procedure for documentation and follow-up.
10. Apply topical ointment if ordered.
11. Cover lightly with an occlusive sterile dressing.
12. Apply cold or warm compresses as indicated (see Table 8-6).
13. Elevate the extremity.
14. Observe regularly for pain, erythema, induration, and necrosis.
15. Documentation of extravasation management:
    a. Date
    b. Time
    c. Needle or catheter size and type
    d. Insertion site
    e. Drug sequence
    f. Approximate amount of drug extravasated
    g. Nursing management of extravasation
    h. Photo documentation
    i. Patient complaints and statements

    j. Appearance of site
    k. Physician notification
    l. Follow-up measures
    m. Nurse's signature

Clinical Alert: The process of tissue destruction resulting from drug extravasation may be subtle and progressive. Initial symptoms include pain or burning at IV site, progressing to erythema, edema, and superficial skin loss. Tissue necrosis may not develop from 1 to 4 weeks after the drug extravasation.

Table 8-6.   Chemotherapeutic vesicant drugs with recommended antidotes

Drug	Antidote
Alkylating agent	Isotonic
Mechlorethamine (Nitrogen Mustard)	Sodium thiosulfate 1/6-molar-4.4 g/10 ml
	Mix 4 ml of 10% sodium thiosulfate with 6 ml sterile water for injection; apply cold compresses
Antibiotics	Hydrocortisone 100 mg/ml
Doxorubicin (Adriamycin) Daunomycin (Cerubidine) Mitomycin C (Mutamycin)	Inject 0.5 ml IV through existing IV line and 0.5 ml sub.q. into extravasated site; apply cold compresses
	Dexamathasone 4 mg/ml
	Inject 0.5 ml IV through existing IV line and 0.5 ml sub.q. into extravasated site; apply cold compresses

Table 8-6. Chemotherapeutic vesicant drugs with recommended antidotes—cont'd

Drug	Antidote
	Alternate protocol
	Topical DMSD 1 to 2 ml of 1 mmol DMSD 50% to 100%
	Apply topically one time at the site; apply cold compresses
Bisantrene	Sodium bicarbonate 1 mEq/ml
	Mix equal parts of sodium bicarbonate with sterile normal saline (1:1 solution); resulting solution is 0.5 mEq/ml
	Inject 2 to 6 ml (1 to 3.0 mEq) IV through existing IV line and sub.q. into the extravasated site; apply cold compresses
Vinca Alkaloids	Hyaluronidase (Wydase) 150 u/ml
Vinblastine (Velban) Vincristine (Oncovin) Vindesine (Eldisine)	Add 1 ml sterile sodium chloride
	Inject 1 to 6 ml (150 to 900 u) sub.q. into the extravasated site with multiple injections; apply warm compresses

Documentation Recommendations

- Site assessment before and after infusion or injection of chemotherapeutic drug
- Establishment of blood return before, during, and after IV and intraarterial infusion of chemotherapy
- Establishment of catheter or device patency before, during, and after infusion of chemotherapy, for example, intraperitoneal, intrathecal
- Patient/family education regarding understanding of chemotherapy protocol—potential side effects and toxicities, self-management of side effects, and schedule of follow-up blood counts, tests, and procedures
- Chemotherapeutic drug, dose, route, and time
- Premedications or postmedications, other infusions, and supplies used for chemotherapy drug regimen
- Any patient complaints of discomfort and symptoms experienced before, during, and after chemotherapeutic infusion

Nursing Diagnoses

- Knowledge deficit, related to chemotherapeutic side effects
- Oral mucous membrane, alteration in, related to side effects of drugs
- Injury, potential for, related to alteration in immune system
- Injury, potential for, related to alteration in clotting factors
- Sexual dysfunction, related to effects of chemotherapeutic drugs (alkylating agents)
- Nutrition, alteration in: less than body requirements related to nausea and vomiting

Patient/Family Teaching for Self-Management

- Assess patient's ability and willingness to learn, availability of caregiver, environment at home, ability to assume self-care, and compliance with treatment regimen.
- Describe purpose, schedule, and procedure of chemotherapeutic regimen.
- Explain to the patient the potential side effects from chemotherapeutic drugs (nausea and vomiting, anorexia, stomatitis, constipation, diarrhea, alopecia, and skin and hemopoietic changes).

- Instruct the patient or the caregiver on self-management interventions specific to each of the side effects.
- Review symptoms such as temperature elevation over 38° C, severe constipation or diarrhea, persistent bleeding from any site, sudden weight gain or loss, shortness of breath, pain not relieved by prescribed medications, and severe nausea and vomiting more than 24 hours after treatment, and reporting of these symptoms promptly to the physician.
- Instruct the patient or the caregiver regarding management of infusion devices of patient receiving chemotherapy in the home.
- Validate aseptic technique and skills of the patient or the caregiver for prescribed self-administration and discontinuation of chemotherapeutic drugs.
- Explain safe handling precautions for administration and disposal of chemotherapy.
- Provide information and list of resources for obtaining, storing, and disposing of drugs and supplies, and schedule of follow-up tests and care.

Home Care Considerations

- Store drugs in a safe, recommended environment, for example, refrigeration, away from sunlight.
- Follow procedures for preparation and administration of chemotherapy as in agency or hospital.
- Record drug, dose, route, and time given in home and provide this information to agency responsible for care management.
- Discard all unused drugs and used supplies into a recommended puncture-proof, leakproof container, and return this container to appropriate agency for disposal.
- Use plastic sheeting to protect bedding or furniture if incontinence is possible.
- Carefully handle linen contaminated from chemotherapeutic drugs and excreta, and wash two times separately from all other linen.
- It is recommended that the patient receive the first dose of the drug(s) in an acute care or outpatient setting.

Clinical Alert: Home care nursing personnel should be alert and prepared for the possible complications of anaphylaxis and drug extravasation; the drugs and supplies necessary to manage these potential complications must be readily available for use.

Pediatric Considerations

- Consider the child's level of cognitive development when preparing him for chemotherapeutic administration.
- Seek to assist in maintaining the child's developmental status and achieving of normal milestones throughout the course of the chemotherapeutic regimen.
- Encourage parents to actively participate in child's care.
- Include the parent in the components of teaching related to potential side effects and toxicities, drug administration schedule, and safe handling measures.
- Anticipate potential side effects of chemotherapeutic drugs and include age, appropriate assessments, and interventions into the nursing management, for example, hair loss, anorexia.
- Instruct the parent regarding safe handling measures for linen contaminated with chemotherapeutic drugs, for example, wear gloves when changing diapers.
- Consider play therapy to minimize distress associated with treatment protocols, for example, intrusive procedures.
- There is potential for increased risk of aspiration in small children resulting from nausea and vomiting; position the child appropriately and monitor the child on scheduled basis.
- Check drug dose calculations and drug reconstitution with another professional to ensure accuracy of dose.
- The child's height and weight will change throughout the course of treatment; recalculate the drug dose based on an accurate height and weight with each course of chemotherapy.
- Keep an accurate, up-to-date, cumulative dose record on all children receiving chemotherapeutic drugs with maximum safe doses.
- Intrathecal dosage may be based on age as estimate of cerebral spinal fluid volume rather than on BSA or body weight.

Chapter
Resource

Safe Handling of Antineoplastic Agents—Process Audit

Agency Name _____

Nurse's Name _____
Monitor's Name _____
Date _____

	Yes	No	NA
Preparation and Administration of Antineoplastic Drugs			
1. Hands are washed before preparing drug.			
2. Eye glasses or goggles are worn during drug preparation.			
3. Eye glasses or goggles are worn during drug administration.			
4. Polyethelene gown is worn during drug preparation.			
5. Polyethelene gown is worn during drug administration.			
6. Gown is changed between patients.			
7. Gown is removed before leaving unit for errands.			
8. Latex gloves are worn during drug preparation.			
9. Latex gloves are worn during drug administration.			
10. Latex gloves are changed approximately every 30 minutes during drug preparation.			
11. Latex gloves are changed approximately every 30 minutes during drug administration.			
12. Luer-Lok fitting syringes are used for drug preparation.			

Continued.

Safe Handling of Antineoplastic Agents—Process Audit—cont'd

	Yes	No	NA
Preparation and Administration of Antineoplastic Drugs			
13. Luer-Lok fitting syringes are used for drug administration.			
14. Chemo-stick pin is used when withdrawing drug from a multi- or single-dose vial.			
15. A sterile alcohol wipe is used when breaking the cap off a glass ampule.			
16. Caution is used when removing air bubbles from filled syringe; sterile alcohol wipe is placed at needle, syringe, or IV tubing tip.			
17. All IV tubings are preprimed and tubing connection is checked for secure fitting of syringe or needle.			
18. Caution is used when inserting needle, syringe, or IV tubing (containing antineoplastic drugs) and when injecting drug into the patient's IV site, for example, Hickman catheter, Port-a-Cath, or heparin lock.			
19. Work area is kept clean and organized.			
Disposal of Antineoplastic Agents/Supplies/Linen/Excreta			
1. Contaminated needles and syringes are disposed intact into chemo waste box.			
2. Gown and gloves are removed and disposed into chemo waste box.			
3. All antineoplastic drug supplies—syringes, IV tubings, IV bags, used alcohol wipes—are disposed into chemo waste box.			
4. Hands are washed after disposing waste products and removing gloves.			
5. Chemo waste box is properly labeled with expiration date of 24 hours or less.			
6. Chemo waste box is properly secured for disposal pickup.			

Disposal of Antineoplastic
Agents/Supplies and Patient Excreta

7. Can discuss appropriate handling of linen
   soiled with chemotherapy spill
8. Can discuss procedure for disposal of patient excreta.

Management of Antineoplastic Drug Spillage

1. Knows placement of and is able to use
   chemo-spill kit.
2. Can briefly state management of antineoplastic drug spill on hard surface, for example, countertop or floor.
3. Can briefly state management of antineoplastic drug spill on soft surface, for example, linen or clothing.
4. Can briefly state management of antineoplastic drug spill on person, for example,
   patient or nurse.
5. Can demonstrate use of eye wash adapters.

Notification Caution Label for Chemotherapy

1. Caution label for chemotherapy is attached to IV solution to remind hospital
   personnel not to alter IV rate and to report
   immediately to unit if there is an IV dis-
   connection or a chemotherapy spillage.

Parenteral nutrition is the IV form of nutritional support. Since this treatment is expensive and can cause significant risks to the patient, IV methods are used only when a catabolic (starvation) state is present or when the patient's digestive system does not function. The goal of parenteral nutrition is to provide all essential nutrients in adequate amounts to sustain an individual in nutritional balance during periods when oral or enteral routes of feeding are impossible or insufficient to meet the patient's needs.

Indications For Parenteral Nutrition

Total parental nutrition (TPN) is used as adjunctive therapy in patients with severe intestinal disease who would otherwise starve (Figure 9-1). Much research, often with conflicting results, has been conducted on the effectiveness of parenteral nutrition as supplemental therapy. Exactly which conditions are improved demonstrably by TPN is controversial. As a rule of thumb, parenteral nutrition is indicated for patients who are severely malnourished and cannot be fed adequately using the oral or enteral route.

The following conditions are often treated with TPN:
1. Gastrointestinal dysfunctions, for example, inflammatory bowel disease, short bowel syndrome, pancreatitis, colitis, obstructive disease, fistulas, radiation enteritis, ileus, or intractable diarrhea
2. Hepatic failure
3. Hypermetabolic states, for example, sepsis, severe burns, long bone fractures
4. Anorexia nervosa
5. Effects of chemotherapy in cancer

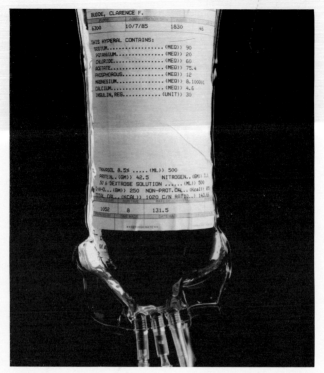

Figure 9-1

17 gauge

Parenteral nutrition infusion.

From Perry AG and Potter PA: Clinical nursing skills and techniques, St Louis, 1986, The CV Mosby Co.

Nutritional Requirements

Both energy and nutrient sources are required by all persons in health and in illness. Without adequate nonprotein calories, the body uses its own protein from muscles, from visceral stores, and from the amino acids provided in the parenteral nutrition solution. An objective of parenteral nutrition is to meet energy needs through nonprotein calorie sources so that the infused amino acids can be directed toward protein synthesis. (Protein breakdown for energy is a catabolic process; protein synthesis is an anabolic process.)

Parenteral nutrition solutions contain energy sources in the forms of dextrose and lipids, as well as nitrogen sources in the form of amino acids, vitamins, and trace elements. The amounts of the various components of parenteral nutrition vary according to patient condition; however, the combinations of components tend to be standard. Each of the basic components of parenteral nutrition is discussed below.

Energy

Energy required by the body for metabolic processes, heat production, and physical activity can be provided by carbohydrates, protein, or fat. Energy needs are met in parenteral nutrition through dextrose (carbohydrate) and lipid (fat) administration. The greater the intake of carbohydrates and fat, the less protein is needed to achieve nitrogen balance. Even though basal levels of glucose and fat are required for normal body processes, there is not a fixed recommendation for the ratio of glucose to fat that should be provided (see Table 9-1 for a summary of the disadvantages of using only dextrose or only fat as the nonnitrogen energy source).

Table 9-1   Disadvantages of either glucose or fat as the sole nonnitrogen energy source in TPN

Glucose	Fat
Increase of basal metabolic rate	Limited elimination capacity
Increased release of catecholamines	Reduced tolerance in prematures
Increased release of insulin	Risk of fat overload
Increased release of glucagon	Immune functions—impairment?
Hyperglycemia	Increased gluconeogenesis—nitrogen losses
Increased CO_2 production	Ketone body formation—acidosis
Essential fatty acid deficiency	
Lipid deposition in the liver	

From Ekman L and Wretlind A: The glucose-lipid ratio in parenteral nutrition, Nutr Support Serv 5[9]:26, 1985.

CNS (Central nervous System)

The energy expenditure of healthy individuals depends mostly on the basal metabolic rate and the level of physical activity. In illness a greater amount of energy is often required because the individual's metabolic rate is increased. For example, prolonged fever increases energy requirements by 7% per Fahrenheit degree and 13% per centigrade degree. A widely used method for calculating resting energy expenditure is the Harris-Benedict equations (see "Chapter Resources"). During illness, caloric (energy) needs vary according to age, sex, height, weight, activity, and the presence of catabolic states such as sepsis, severe injuries, and burns.

Carbohydrates

Carbohydrates, in the form of glucose, are the major energy source for humans and are the only energy source for the central nervous system (CNS). The CNS requires about 150 g of glucose per day. Dextrose is the least expensive source of glucose and is available in concentrations of 5% to 70% dextrose in water. Concentrated dextrose is the primary calorie source in TPN.

Fat emulsion

Fat is the chief storage source of energy in the body. Fat emulsions, also called lipid solutions, provide a concentrated source of energy during parenteral nutrition. Fat emulsions are available in 10% and 20% concentrations. Fat may be administered to provide 40% to 60% of total daily calories. Only 140 calories is provided by 1 L of 5% dextrose in water solution, although 1100 calories is provided by 1 L of 10% fat.

In addition, lipids are a source of essential fatty acids and thus can prevent or correct fatty acid deficiencies. Since use of fatty acids can provide fuel for most tissues, glucose can then be made available for use by the CNS, and protein for anabolic processes.

Protein

A compromised patient experiences a greater improvement in weight gain and wound healing with the use of IV amino acids than with the use of only IV dextrose. While protein can provide energy, the continued breakdown of protein for energy adversely affects body functioning, growth, and tissue repair. Enough protein must be administered to replace essential amino acids; otherwise the body will convert its own protein to glucose to meet energy requirements. If body protein is converted to glucose, the patient experiences a persistent loss of protein primarily from muscle tissue, causing a negative nitrogen balance. Since excess protein is metabolized and not stored in the body, maintenance of adequate protein stores is a major objective of nutritional support.

Protein is provided in parenteral nutrition in the form of amino acids, but optimal amino acid levels have not been established. Available preparations containing varying amounts of essential and nonessential amino acids are available in concentrations of 3.5% to 10%. Since the nitrogen from protein metabolization is excreted principally through urine, nitrogen loss is measured through urine sampling. Because a small amount of nitrogen is lost through hair, skin, saliva, and stool, a correction factor for these losses is added to the Harris-Benedict equation. (See "Chapter Resources.")

Vitamins

Vitamins function as essential cofactors in a number of enzymatic processes and cannot be manufactured within the body. Although actual IV vitamin requirements are unknown, IV requirements are considered greater than oral requirements because of increased renal excretion and adsorption of vitamins to IV bags and tubings. Other factors considered in calculating vitamin dosages are the degree of stress experienced by the patient and the extent of depletion present.

Vitamins are classified as either water soluble or fat soluble. Water-soluble vitamins are vitamin C, folate, and the B-complex vitamins: thiamine, riboflavin, niacin, pyridoxine, cobalamin, and biotin. Fat-soluble vitamins are A, D, E, and K. Vitamin K is not included in most commercially prepared IV vitamin solutions because of possible adverse effects in patients taking oral anticoagulants.

Trace Elements

Trace elements are those elements present in the body in extremely small amounts. Like vitamins, trace elements must be provided in long-term parenteral therapy for normal metabolism to take place. All trace elements participate in enzymatic reactions and act as cofactors for other metabolic processes. Currently 15 trace elements have been identified; however, the exact requirements for each element are unknown. Among those thought to be essential are iron, iodine, cobalt, zinc, copper, chromium, and manganese. Commercially prepared trace element combinations are available.

Vitamin	Function	Deficiency
Vitamin A	Retinal function Prevents night blindness Bone metabolism	Night blindness Reproductive failure
Vitamin C	Wound healing	Scurvy
Vitamin D	Calcium absorption	Rickets
Vitamin E	Protects cellular membrane Prevents oxidation of vitamins A and C	May contribute to hemolytic anemia and liver necrosis
Vitamin K	Prothrombin formation	Prolonged clotting time and bleeding
Iron	Oxygen transport	Anemia
Zinc	Cofactor of many enzymes	Poor wound healing Growth retardation Diminished taste and smell Gonadal dysfunction
Copper	Hemoglobin synthesis	Associated with neutropenia
Calcium	Bone metabolism Neuromuscular function	Osteoporosis Tetany
Magnesium	Bone metabolism Neuromuscular function	Neuromuscular irritability
Phosphate	Found in bone Serum levels regulated by kidney reabsorption	Skeletal and cardiac muscle dysfunction
Potassium	Principal cation in ICF Neuromuscular function	Critical cardiac dysrhythmias
Sodium	Principal cation in ECF Regulates acid-base balance Neuromuscular function	Alteration in balance of ICF and ECF

Vitamin	Function	Deficiency
Sulfate	Protein synthesis	Wasting
Iodine	Thyroid function	Hypothyroidism

Fluids and Electrolytes

Because they are determined by the patient's condition, fluid and electrolyte needs vary widely. Fluid needs vary when a condition causing fluid loss, fever, or renal or cardiac impairment is present. The amount of water provided in parenteral fluids depends on the patient's fluid needs. Water needs are determined by closely monitoring the patient's weight and intake and output. The greater the dextrose and amino acid concentration of the infusion, the less water will be delivered. For example, 70% dextrose solutions are used when fluid restriction is desired.

Electrolytes are adjusted by the physician according to serum levels. Additional potassium may be needed as glucose is metabolized.

Other Additives

Sometimes other agents are added to parenteral nutrition fluids. Medications such as regular insulin, heparin, and corticosteroids may be prescribed by the physician when a patient need exists.

Nutritional Assessment

Assessing the nutritional status of the patient is important when deciding whether parenteral nutrition is necessary and also when monitoring therapy. A diet history, anthropometric measurements, and laboratory tests are all used in the assessment. Each method currently used to assess the extent of malnutrition experienced by a patient has limitations. Currently there is no single, best test for evaluating nutritional status, since many factors influence an individual's nutritional condition. Ultrasonography, magnetic resonance imaging, and computed tomography scans are among the assessment tools that are the focus of current nutritional research.

Nutritional Status Indicators	Comments
Diet history	Includes 24-hour recall, food allergies or intolerances, appetite, chewing and swallowing difficulties, changes in food intake
Height and weight	Compared to standard height and weight tables; actual body weight is calculated as a percentage of ideal weight
Basal energy expenditure (BEE)	Estimate of the energy requirements at rest (Harris-Benedict equation)
Anthropometric measurements	Measurements of the midarm circumference, skinfold thickness, and arm muscle area are compared to standard values as a way of inferring patient body mass
Creatinine/height index	Indicates status of muscle stores in patients with normal renal function; creatinine is released from muscle at a constant rate in proportion to muscle mass; patient's index is compared to standards to determine the degree of impairment 5% to 15%—mild impairment 15% to 30%—moderate impairment greater than 30%—severe impairment
Serum transferrin	Indicates a combination of protein depletion and iron deficiency 150 to 200 mg/dl—mild depletion 100 to 150 mg/dl—moderate depletion less than 30 mg/dl—severe depletion
Albumin levels	Indirect measures of visceral protein mass; low values are associated with reduced dietary protein or excessive losses; does not reflect immediate changes—20-day half-life
Prealbumin	Short half-life; provides an analysis of protein changes during previous two days; 17 to 42 mg/dl—normal

Nutritional Status Indicators	Comments
Total lymphocyte count	Used for screening immune function; obtained from the CBC and differential 1200 to 2000/mm^3—mild depletion 800 to 1200/mm^3—moderate depletion less than 800/mm^3—severe depletion
T-cell counts	Measure cellular and humoral immune function; normal T_4 to T_8 ratio is 2
Skin antigen tests	Commonly used antigens include purified protein derivative (PPD), streptokinase-streptodornase (SKSD), *Candida,* mumps, and *Trichophyton;* positive response if 5 mm induration at 72 hours; used to measure response to nutritional therapy
Nitrogen balance	Nitrogen is an essential element of protein required for tissue building; measured as the total nitrogen excreted in urine, plus a correction factor for unmeasured losses, minus the total nitrogen consumed in the form of protein; *positive* nitrogen balance exists when nitrogen intake is greater than nitrogen loss; *negative* nitrogen balance is found in persons who are inadequately fed relative to protein needs: protein is broken down to meet their metabolic needs, and thus these persons excrete more nitrogen than they take in

Administration of Parenteral Nutrition

Central Venous Administration

Parenteral nutrition may be administered through a peripheral vein or through a central vein depending on the osmolality of the solution. Dextrose concentrations greater than 12.5% need to be given through a large central vein, usually the subclavian. (See Chapter 3 for guidelines on managing central venous catheters.)

Peripheral Parenteral Nutrition

Parenteral nutrition may be administered through peripheral veins as maintenance nutrition for patients who are nutritionally compromised and unable to receive sufficient calories through oral or enteral routes. Maintenance parenteral nutrition is administered both preoperatively and postoperatively to surgical patients with a nutritional deficit in an effort to minimize the adverse effects of malnutrition.

The major disadvantage of the peripheral route of administration is that a large fluid volume per gram of dextrose is required to deliver acceptable osmolalities. For example, a 10% dextrose solution provides only 340 calories/liter. To deliver 2000 calories each day would require 6 liters of 10% dextrose. Additional calories are added through the administration of fat emulsions. A 10% fat emulsion provides 550 calories per 500 ml of solution. Another disadvantage is thrombophlebitis, which is a frequent complication of peripheral parenteral nutrition because the solutions are irritating to the patient's veins. *ween slowly*

Total Parenteral Nutrition

Total parenteral nutrition (TPN) is administered over an extended period to maintain or increase a patient's lean body mass. Since hypertonic concentrations of dextrose and amino acids are necessary to provide adequate energy without fluid overload, a large central vein is required to provide rapid dilution of the fluid.

Initiating therapy

To ensure glucose tolerance, TPN infusions are initially increased at a rate that allows endogenous insulin production to handle the extra glucose load. Until the patient is in a stable state, daily weights, intake and output, blood glucose tests, electrolytes, and all other laboratory reports require close monitoring.

Discontinuing therapy

There are many methods recommended for discontinuing parenteral nutrition. Tapering of the infusion rate over at least several hours is usually recommended to prevent severe hypoglycemia. *no more than 24 hrs.*

Total Nutritional Admixture or 3-in-1 Admixture

Total nutritional admixtures (TNAs) combine a 24-hour supply of parenteral nutrition in a 3-liter container. Research on the chemical stability of TPN solutions, growth of microorganisms, and compounding techniques has led to procedures that make TNAs safe and convenient. Lipids are mixed with the dextrose and amino acid solution in the pharmacy. TNA solutions are solid white and have a nonreflecting surface making precipitation difficult to observe. This form of TPN is usually reserved for patients in a stable state, since the components are adjusted only once daily.

Advantages of TNA

1. Risk of contamination is reduced, since the TPN system is manipulated only once every 24 hours.
2. Fat emulsions do not need to be piggybacked.
3. Pharmacy compounding time is reduced, since only one bag is prepared every 24 hours.
4. Nursing time associated with setting up infusions is reduced.
5. Fewer supplies are required.

Disadvantages of TNA

1. It is costly to adjust components of TNA more frequently than every 24 hours, since a new admixture is required.
2. Some infusion pumps do not accurately deliver the large admixture volume.

Equipment considerations

1. TNA solutions cannot be filtered with standard IV tubing filters. Where agency policy requires the filtering of all solutions, a large (1.2 μm) filter, not a 0.22 μm filter, should be used.
2. Verify that infusion pump can deliver this product accurately.

Clinical Alert: Examine TNA admixtures before hanging for evidence of an unstable solution. Unstable solutions have small, clear, or slightly yellow pools of oil floating on the surface.

Considerations When Administering Parenteral Nutrition

1. If possible, do not use the parenteral nutrition catheter for other purposes. If using a multilumen catheter, dedicate one lumen only to the TPN solution. Never use this lumen to administer piggyback medications, blood, or blood products. Do not draw laboratory samples from the TPN lumen, and do not use this lumen for measuring central venous pressures.
2. Refrigerate admixed solutions at 4° C. Remove solutions from refrigeration approximately 30 minutes before use.

3. Perform additional admixture of solutions only in consultation with the pharmacist and never at the bedside, since microbial and particulate contamination is a primary concern in TPN.
4. Do not allow TNA bags (3-in-1) to hang longer than 24 hours.
5. Suspect catheter sepsis if a previously afebrile patient has a fever. Notify the physician.
6. Solutions that have changed color are unacceptable for infusion, since color changes result from decomposition of carbohydrates and amino acids during long-term storage.
7. Follow strict aseptic technique at all times when handling the catheter, dressing, tubing, or solution.
8. If the infusion falls behind schedule, do not attempt to catch up. Readjust the rate to the prescribed infusion rate.

Considerations When Administering Fat Emulsions

1. Use unfiltered tubing, since the fat molecules are too large to pass through a filter smaller than 1.2 μm.
2. Monitor blood lipid levels and liver function tests.
3. When administering lipids by the piggyback method, use the Y-tube injection site closest to the catheter hub.
4. Do not use the solution if oil has separated.
5. Administer fat emulsions by peripheral vein, since the solution is isotonic.

Information To Report To The Physician

1. Blood glucose levels above 200 mg/dl
2. Hypoglycemia—blood glucose levels below 60 mg/dl
3. Urine glucose level above 1+ on test strip
4. Abnormal electrolyte results

Complications of Parenteral Nutrition

Many serious complications may occur during parenteral nutrition. Contamination of some part of the infusion system is a major concern. A break in sterile technique at any point during manufacture, compounding, or infusion may cause contamination (Figure 9-2). Avoidance of contamination requires strict observance of sterile technique. Complications of parenteral nutrition are provided below.

Type	Examples
Catheter	Technical problems at the time of insertion: pneumothorax, hemothorax Problems after placement: thrombus formation, dislodgement, fibrin clot formation, vessel problems, and catheter tear (See Chapter 3)
Infusion equipment	Separation of tubing junctions; malfunction of infusion pump
Metabolic	Hypoglycemia or hyperglycemia, other blood chemistry abnormalities, vitamin and mineral imbalances, hematologic complications

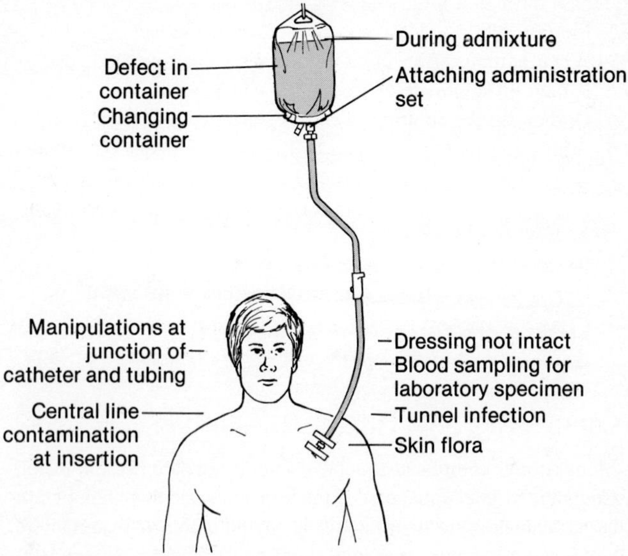

Figure 9-2

Sites for contamination of parenteral nutrition system.
From Williams WW: Infection control during parenteral nutrition therapy, J Parenter Enteral Nutr 9:736, 1985.

Documentation Recommendations

Documentation of the patient's and caregiver's ability to perform all procedures and their understanding of troubleshooting measures, potential complications, and appropriate interventions is essential. Points to include in documentation are the following:

- Site assessment before and during the infusion
- Observation of catheter or device patency before, during, and after infusion
- Components of parenteral nutrition solution
- Infusion rate and any equipment used for regulation
- All supplies used; date and time of tubing changes
- Any complaints of discomfort and symptoms experienced before, during, or after infusion; action taken to correct problems
- Patient weight; fluid intake and output record
- All patient and caregiver education for self-management

Nursing Diagnoses

- Knowledge deficit regarding home care management of nutrition and venous catheter
- Nutrition, altered: less than body requirements, related to inadequate intake or absorption of foods
- Infection, potential for, related to high dextrose content of parenteral solution, break in sterile technique when managing catheter, or contamination of supplies
- Self-concept, disturbance in: body image, related to placement of vascular access device
- Coping, ineffective family: related to inadequate financial resources, family role changes, or stressors associated with parenteral nutrition management.

Support Needs of Patients and Caregivers

The disruption of normal eating patterns and the intensity of long-term self-management required of persons who need parenteral nutrition place significant pressure on the patient and the family. Dependence on TPN leads to feelings of loss of control over many aspects of normal daily life and often progresses to periods of depression.

Food and eating are associated with many positive feelings such as security, acceptance, and belonging. Disruption of normal eating patterns, particularly over long periods of time, removes a major source of pleasure for the patients. If a patient is not eating, he is deprived of the sense of taste and of participating fully in social occasions involving food. The patient and family should be assisted in developing alternatives to food-related functions and in discovering ways of participating in social events designed around food.

Support and encouragement from the family are required as new procedures are learned and as adaptations in daily schedules are made around infusions. Encourage patient and family discussion of questions and feelings with the nursing staff and the physician. Acknowledge that patient and family feelings and concerns are commonly experienced by persons who require parenteral nutrition; occasional feelings of discouragement are to be expected. Reassure them that help is available when it is needed, and that they will be able to readjust successfully and return to normal activities.

Clinical Alert: Frequent mouth care such as brushing teeth and using mouthwash and lip gloss is often helpful for the patient who is not eating. If the patient is allowed to eat but is experiencing anorexia, encourage small, frequent meals with others present.

Patient/Family Teaching for Self-Management

Extensive, formalized education is required for successful self-management of parenteral nutrition. Good communication of every aspect of management is required. Supervised practice with return demonstration is as important as written and visual materials that are easily understood by the patient and family. Initial teaching of both the patient and caregiver should take place in the hospital and be completed in the home. If the patient has difficulty reading, consider making an audiotape describing each procedure in a step-by-step fashion.

Hospital-Based Teaching

1. Assess ability and willingness to learn, availability of the caregiver, home environment, ability to assume self-care, and compliance with treatment regimen.
2. Describe purpose and procedures for the parenteral nutrition regimen.

3. Explain and demonstrate aseptic technique; stress that sterile technique is essential, and be consistent in all demonstrations and instructions to the patient and family; allow patients and families to handle equipment as much as possible.
4. Break each procedure into small tasks and guide the patient through each task; have the patient and the caregiver talk each other through each procedure to enhance learning.
5. Validate aseptic technique and skills of both the patient and the caregiver for initiation and discontinuation of therapy.
6. Instruct the patient and caregiver in signs, symptoms, and self-management interventions specific to each complication, for example, lethargy, fluid retention, increased urine output, catheter complications.
7. Instruct the patient and caregiver in the management of infusion devices.
8. Provide information and list of resources for obtaining home-care services.
9. Ensure that follow-up care has been scheduled.

Home-Based Teaching

Since home and hospital environments are different, the patient and family need assistance transferring information learned in the hospital to the home setting. Written materials are required, and checklists should be provided for each procedure to be performed by the patient and for all necessary supplies. Equipment and supplies used in the hospital often are different from those available through the home-care agency; specific instructions will be needed. Provide the patient with telephone numbers for 24-hour assistance.

1. Teach use of all home equipment; include troubleshooting tips for infusion pump alarms and malfunctions.
2. Validate aseptic technique and skills.
3. Evaluate home refrigeration and supply storage areas.
4. Teach the patient and caregiver how to order supplies.
5. Advise on disposal of used supplies.
6. Review symptoms and implications of infection and all other complications; ensure that what is to be done in case of a complication is known by both the patient and the family.
7. Provide listing of emergency phone numbers.

Home Care Considerations

Medical stability, a motivated patient and family, and comprehensive agency support are required for successful home parenteral nutrition. Home TPN is scheduled usually over 10 to 14 hours during the night. This allows the patient to assume a more normal daytime schedule.

Although equipment needs are similar at home and in the hospital, pumps with readouts that can be read in the dark minimize sleep disturbances. Poles that can be pushed easily over carpet also allow greater mobility for the patient.

Patients should be taught to check regularly their weight and temperature. The patient or caregiver should be instructed how to read accurately both the scale and the thermometer. They should be provided with a record to document weights and temperature readings.

Patients and families need assistance with organizing and storing supplies. Optimally, a home visit is made by the home health nurse before the patient's dismissal to prepare for the patient's homecoming. If the home health referral agency is in an outreach area, copies of all protocols help diminish confusion and disparities between services.

Pediatric Considerations

Pediatric parenteral nutrition is highly specialized and requires the fulfillment of both growth and maintenance needs. When parenteral nutritional support is managed in the home environment, parents require significant instruction and support.

Chapter
Resources

Calculations Frequently Used in Nutritional Assessment

Harris-Benedict equation

Female: BEE = 655 + (9.6 × Wt.) + (1.7 × Ht.) − (4.7 × Age)

Male: BEE = 66 + (13.7 × Wt.) + (5 × Ht.) − (6.8 × Age)

where *BEE* stands for basal energy expenditure, *Wt.* stands for patient weight in kilograms, and *Ht.* is for patient height in centimeters.

Weight should be calculated according to the ideal body weight when the patient is in a state of starvation so that protein stores can be replenished.

Often an additional calculation is added to estimate activity, severity of illness, and other related disease states that may increase energy requirements. This requires a subjective evaluation of patient stress. This correction factor is listed below:

Low stress: 1.3 × BEE

Moderate stress: 1.5 × BEE

Severe stress: 2.0 × BEE

Percentage of weight loss = number of kilograms lost/usual weight

Total lymphocyte count = WBC × percentage of lymphocytes/ 100

Creatinine/height index = actual urinary creatinine/ideal urinary creatinine × 100

Nitrogen balance = nitrogen intake − nitrogen excretion

= protein intake in grams/6.25 = (UUN+4)

where UUN is the urine urea nitrogen.

Base Solutions	Bottle # __ Infuse Over __ Hours		Bottle # __ Infuse Over __ Hours	
Aminosyn 3.5% M	ml		ml	
Nephramine	ml		ml	
Dextrose 70% & water	ml		ml	
Freamine 11 8.5%	ml		ml	
Dextrose 50% & water	ml		ml	
Dextrose 20% & water	ml		ml	
Dextrose 10% & water	ml		ml	
Electrolytes & Vitamins				
Regular insulin	Units		Units	
Heparin	Units		Units	
Potassium acetate	mEq		mEq	
Potassium chloride	mEq		mEq	
Potassium phosphate	mM		mM	
Sodium acetate	mEq		mEq	
Sodium chloride	mEq		mEq	
Sodium phosphate	mM		mM	
Calcium gluconate	mEq		mEq	
Magnesium sulfate	mEq		mEq	
Hyperlyte	ml		ml	
Multiple vitamin infusion	ml		ml	
Folic acid	mg		mg	
Vitamin K	mg		mg	
Vitamin B-12	mcg		mcg	
Totals				

Date _____ Time ___ Dr. _____
                                    Physician's Signature

Bottle # __ Infuse Over __ Hours		Pharmacy Use
ml		
ml		
ml		
ml		
ml		
ml		
ml		
Units		
Units		
mEq		
mEq		
mM		
mEq		
mEq		
mM		
mEq		
mEq		
ml		
ml		
mg		
mg		
mcg		

Home Care Parenteral Nutrition Weekly Log

Dates:	M	T	W	T	F	S	S	Remarks
TPN completed								
Daily heparin flush								
Daily dressing change								
Daily catheter cap change								
Weight as ordered								
Temperature as ordered								
Blood glucose AM								
Blood glucose PM								
Urine glucose (if applicable)								
Daily tubing change								
TPN started								
Meal(s) eaten daily (1) (2) (3)								
Bowel movements								

Appendix

Use of Nursing Diagnoses with Sample Charting

Infusion Guidelines	Notes
Date Time 1/88 0900 Procedure	1000 ml D5 0.45 NS with 40 mEq KCl at 125 ml/hr using macrodrop tubing initiated. Insertion site right cephalic vein without redness or discomfort.
Fluid volume, alteration in, related to intestinal surgical procedure.	Postoperative day (3) right colectomy.
1100	Urine volume from 0700 to 1100 is 250 ml. Bowel sounds active in all four abdominal quadrants. Abdomen palpated; soft distention noted.
1500	Urine volume from 1100 to 1500 is 1050 ml. Expelling flatus at intervals. IV fluids continue at 125 ml/hr. Physician notified of increased urinary output. (Nurse's name)

Venipuncture	Notes
Date Time 1/88 0830 Procedure	Peripheral IV site established in right cephalic vein using 20-gauge 1½ in Angiocath. Sterile technique used and catheter secured according to policy. 1000 ml D5 0.45 NS with 40 mEq KCl infusing at 125 ml/hr.

Venipuncture	Notes
Anxiety related to invasive procedure.	States "this is the first time I've had an IV and I'm nervous." Explained the procedure to the patient. Coached in deep breathing exercise and instructed to focus attention on the picture on center wall during venipuncture stick. (Nurse's name)

Central Venous Catheters	Notes
Date Time 1/88 1000 Procedure	Access of Port-A-Cath, sterile technique used. Huber needle 19-gauge, 1½ in 90 degree inserted, good blood return, flushed with 10 ml NS, then connected to 1000 ml D5 NS at 125 ml/hr.
Skin integrity, impairment of: potential at placement site.	Transparent dressing intact over needle site. Placement site without redness and tenderness.
Injury, potential for, related to catheter occlusion.	IV fluids discontinued, Port-A-Cath system flushed with 10 ml NS, then heparin 5 ml (100 μ/ml) as needle was removed from the portal septum leaving a heparin lock. (Nurse's name)

Calculations for IV Therapy

Nursing diagnosis for patient care does not relate to this chapter.

IV Fluids	Notes
	See "Infusion Guidelines."

Date Time	
1/88 1530	
Procedure	

Fluid volume deficit: potential, related to excessive fluid loss from surgical procedure.	IV fluids 1000 ml D5 0.45 NS, with 40 mEq KCl increased to 150 ml/hr. Insertion site without redness. No complaints of discomfort at IV site or right arm. (Nurse's name)

IV Medication Administration	Notes

Date Time	
1/88 1300	
Procedure	Discontinued D5 0.45 NS IV solution, 600 ml absorbed. Replaced with heparin infusion (20,000 μ/500 ml) at rate of 600 μ/hr. IV site 12 hours old and no erythema or edema noted.

Injury, potential for, related to administration of IV medication.	Placed on infusion pump at rate of 15 ml/hr.

Blood Administration	Notes

Date Time	
1/88 1000	
Procedure	BP 112/72, P 108, R 20, T 98.4 as baseline vital signs. 10 units pooled random platelets initiated. (ID #02 G 54496, O positive), via Y-set IV tubing with 100 ml normal saline bag for flushing of multilumen subclavian catheter. ID numbers on donor unit and patient bracelet verified by L. Borg, RN and S. Miles, RN.

Blood Administration	Notes
1030 Fluid volume deficit: potential, related to loss of blood volume.	No active bleeding at this time from central line exit site: nose bleed diminished 2 cm diameter pinkish red fluid on tissue. BP 114/76, P 112, R 18, T 98. No complaints of discomfort, e.g., shortness of breath, chills, or urticaria.
1100	Bleeding from nose has ceased. BP 116/80, P 116, R 20, T 98.2. Platelet transfusion is completed. Time, date, ID number, and signature completed on transfusion record and record returned to blood bank.
1110 Injury, potential for, related to catheter occlusion.	Subclavian catheter flushed with 2.5 ml normal saline, then tubing disconnected from catheter. Catheter lumen heparin locked with 2.5 ml heparin (100 μ/ml).
1200	Blood sample for platelet count drawn and sent to lab. (Nurse's name)

Chemotherapy	Notes
Date Time 1/88 1030 Procedure	Premedicated with metoclopramide (Reglan) 50 mg IV, dexamethasone (Decadron) 20 mg IV, and Benadryl 50 mg IV prior to administration of Cytoxan 500 mg, Adriamycin 75 mg, vincristine 1.5 mg. Chemotherapy drugs given through a free-flowing IV of normal saline into peripheral site (20-gauge 1½ inch

Chemotherapy	Notes
	Angiocath) in right hand. IV site without swelling or redness. No complaint of burning or pain before, during, or after drug administration. Good blood return obtained throughout the procedure.
Knowledge deficit related to chemotherapy side effects.	Discussion of potential side effects (nausea, hair loss, and tingling of fingers and toes) reviewed with patient. Written materials regarding drugs, potential side effects, and self-management interventions given to patient and spouse. Instructed patient to drink one glass of liquid per hour, eat light meals for today, and empty bladder at least every 4 hours times 24 hours. Patient or spouse to notify physician after discharge if temperature is over 38° C, or persistent nausea. Appointment for lab next Friday. States understanding of side effects, self-management interventions, and pertinent instructions for next 48 hours. (Nurse's name)

Parenteral Nutrition	Notes
Date Time 1/88 2100 Procedure	Parenteral infusion initiated after verifying admixture with prescribed physician order. TPN solution aseptically connected to Groshong catheter. Infusion pump rate set at 200 ml/hr.

Parenteral Nutrition	Notes
2130 Self-concept, disturbance in: body image, related to placement of vascular access device.	Patient states she is concerned about summertime clothing and has ceased activities she normally pursued. Feels embarrassed when disrobing in locker room because of external catheter. Discussed coiling and taping catheter inside bra to secure placement and suggestions given for clothing styles. Discussed feelings at length about these issues. She will try suggestions and share results at next clinic appointment. (Nurse's name)

Bibliography

Infusion Guidelines

Adams SD and others: Inline filtration and infusion phlebitis, Heart Lung 15:2, 1986.

Centers for Disease Control: Recommendations for prevention of HIV transmission in health care settings, MMWR 36[25]:6-18, 1987.

Falchuk L: Microparticulate induced phlebitis, N Engl J Med 312:78-82, 1985.

Gurevich I: Are in-line filters worth the price?, Nursing 16:42-43, 1986.

Intravenous Nursing Society: Intravenous nursing standards of practice, Philadelphia, 1981, JB Lippincott Co.

Nelson R: Keeping air out of IV lines, Nursing 16:57-59, 1986.

Phelps SJ and others: Risk factors affecting infiltration of peripheral venous lines in infants, J Pediatr 111[3]:384-389, 1987.

Venipuncture

Burrows CW: Toward making better IV needle selections, Nursing 14:32-33, 1984.

Fay MJ: The special challenges of pediatric IVs, Dim of Crit Care Nursing 2[1]:23-29, 1983.

Feldstein A: Detect phlebitis and infiltration before they harm your patient, Nursing 16[1]:44-48, 1986

Infiltrating IVs and nurses' negligence, Regan Rep Nurs Law 26[8]:2, 1986.

Jones S: New IV catheters that can do it all, RN 48[2]:20-23, 1985.

Milliam DA: Performing IV procedures like an expert, Nurs Life 6[2]:33-40, 1986.

Milliam DA: Sharpen your drawing skills, Nursing 17[12]:56-58, 1987.

Milliam DA: Tips for improving your venipuncture techniques, Nursing 17[6]:46-49, 1986.

Central Venous Catheters

Bagnall H and Ruccione K: Experience with a totally implanted venous access device in children with malignant disease, Oncol Nurs Forum 14[5]:51-56, 1987.

Cunliffe MT and Polomano RS: How to clear catheter clots with urokinase, Nursing 16:40-43, 1986.

Curnow A and others: Urokinase therapy for Silastic catheter–induced intravascular thrombi in infants and children, Arch Surg 120:1237-1240, 1985.

Ford R: History and organization of the Seattle area, Hickman Catheter Committee, NITA 8:123-135, 1985.

Gililisco PA and Zenowich D: Blood-drawing from central venous catheters using a click-lock vacutainer assembly, Pharmacy Pract News 5:17, 1986.

Groshong CV: Acute care catheter, Salt Lake City, Utah, 1987, Catheter Tech Corp.

Hagle ME: Implantable devices for chemotherapy: access and delivery, Semin Oncol Nurs 3[2]:96-105, 1987.

Hughes CB and Bryant JK: The use of multi-lumen catheters in acute leukemia patients, NITA 7:484-486, 1984.

Kilbride SS: A patient's guide to the implanted port, Oncol Nurs Forum, 13[2]:83-85, 1986.

Moore CL and others: Nursing care and management of venous access ports, Oncol Nurs Forum 13[2]:35-39, 1986.

Nursing Protocol, Port-A-Cath, Pharmacia Deltec, Inc, St Paul, Minn, 1986.

Raaf JH: Results from use of 826 vascular access devices in cancer patients, Cancer 55:1312-1321, 1985.

Simon RC: Small gauge central venous catheters and right atrial catheters, Semin Oncol Nurs 3[2]:87-95, 1987.

Slater HS and others: Experience with long-term outpatient venous access utilizing percutaneously placed silicone elastomer catheters, Cancer 56:2074-2077, 1985.

Strum S and others: Improved methods for venous access: the Port-A-Cath, a totally implanted catheter system, J Clin Oncol 4:596-603, 1986.

Thomas MH and others: How to repair cracks, holes, and tears in central venous catheters, Nursing 17:49-54, 1987.

Warren J: The multi-lumen subclavian catheter, a new answer to an old problem, NITA 8:154-156, 1985.

Calculations for IV Therapy

Hahn AB and others: Mosby's pharmacology in nursing, St Louis, 1986, CV Mosby Co, pp. 98-100.

Lowe J and Fears M: Nomograms shortcuts to accuracy, Focus Crit Care 13[3]:36-40, 1986.

Northridge JA: Calculating IV medications with confidence, Nursing 17:55-59, 1987.

Sackheim GI and Robins L: Programmed mathematics for nurses, ed 6, New York, 1987, Macmillan Publishing Co.

Thwing CJ: Calculating infusion drips—there is an easier way, Crit Care Nurs 4:11, 1984.

Intravenous Fluids

Austin C and others: Water: guidelines for nutritional support, Nutr Support Serv 6[9]:27-29, 1986.

Felver L: Understanding the electrolyte maze, AJN 80:1591-95, 1980.

Folk-Lighty M: Solving the puzzles of patient's fluid imbalances, Nursing 14[2]:34-41, 1984.

Gennari FJ: Serum osmolality: uses and limitations, N Engl J Med 310[2]:102-105, 1984.

Johnston ID: Effects of changes in endocrine function on water and electrolyte metabolism, World J Surg 7[5]:559-603, 1983.

Keithley JK: What's behind that IV line?, Nursing 12[3]:33-45, 1982.

Mascaro J: Managing IV therapy in the home, Nursing 16[5]:50-51, 1986.

Thoren L and others: Intraoperative fluid therapy, World J Surg 7[5]:581-589, 1983.

Wiseman M: Setting standards for home IV therapy, AJN 85:421-423, 1985.

IV Medication Administration

Akers MJ: Current problems and innovations in intravenous drug delivery, Am J Hosp Pharm 44:2528-2529, 1987.

Beumont E: IV infusion pumps, Nurs Manage 18[9]:26-32, 1987.

Burman R: IV bolus: effective but potentially hazardous, Crit Care Nurs 6[1]:22-28, 1986.

Davis NM: Learning from mistakes, Nursing 17:84-91, 1987.

Gorski LA: Effective teaching of home IV therapy, Home Health Nurse 5[5]:10-18, 1987.

Henrietta G: Lab tests you can't overlook, Nursing 17:56-59, 1987.

Hull RL: Prospective changes in drug administration, Nursing 17:55-57, 1987.

Kasmer RJ and others: Home parenteral antibiotic therapy, Home Health Nurse 5[1]:12-18, 1987.

Leff RD: Features of IV devices and equipment that affect IV drug delivery, Am J Hosp Pharm 44:2530-2533, 1987

Mioduszewski J and others: Ambulatory infusion pumps: a practical view at an alternative approach, Semin Oncol Nurs 3[2]:106-111, 1987.

Motz-Harding E and others: Mixing IV drugs thoroughly, Nursing 17:62-64, 1985.

Nahata MC: Effect of IV drug delivery systems on pharmacokinetic monitoring, Am J Hosp Pharm 44:2538-2542, 1987.

Olson C and others: Amphotericin B extravasation, NITA 8:299-300, 1985.

Parker WA: Physical compatibility of critical care medications: what is known?, Crit Care Nurs 4:70-74, 1984.

Randall BJ: Reacting to anaphylaxis, Nursing 16:34-39, 1986.

Rapp RP: Considering product features and costs in selecting a system for intermittent IV drug delivery, Am J Hosp Pharm 44:2533-2538, 1987.

Rehm SJ: Home intravenous antibiotic therapy, Cleve Clin Q 52:333-338, 1985.

Rimar JM: Guidelines for the intravenous administration of medications used in pediatrics, MCN 12:322-340, 1987.

Schad RF: Patient teaching program for home intravenous antimicrobial therapy, Am J Hosp Pharm 43:372-375, 1986.

Treloar D: Cephalosporins: the third generation, RN 49:28-29, 1986.

Zenk K: Administering IV antibiotics to children, Nursing 16:50-52, 1986.

Zenk K: Intravenous drug delivery in infants with limited IV access and fluid restriction, Am J Hosp Pharm 44:2542-2545, 1987.

Epidural Pain Management

Baggerly J: Epidural catheters for pain management: the nurse's role, J Neuro Sci Nurs 18:290-295, 1986.

Coombs DW: Continuous intraspinal morphine analgesia for relief of cancer pain, Etna Village, NH, 1986, Inovasions, Inc.

Coombs DW and others: Outcomes and complications of continuous intraspinal narcotic analgesia for cancer pain control, J Clin Oncol 2:1414-1419, 1984.

Coombs DW and others: Relief of continuous chronic pain by intraspinal narcotics infusion via an implanted reservoir, JAMA 250:2336-2339, 1983.

Coyle N and others: A model of continuity of care for cancer patients with pain and neuro-oncologic complications, Cancer Nurs 8:111-119, 1985.

Dunajcik L: Controlling the dangers of epidural analgesia, RN 1:40-47, 1988.

Jernigan DK: Home management of epidural catheters for pain control, Caring 85-91, Oct 1986.

Maglia RA: Ambulatory epidural morphine therapy, Hosp Pharm 22:707-708, 1987.

Pagean MG and others: New analgesic therapy relieves cancer pain without over-sedation, Nursing 15:46-49, April 1985.

Paice JA: Intrathecal morphine infusion for intractable cancer pain: a new use for implanted pumps, Oncol Nurs Forum 13:41-47, 1986.

Payne R: Novel routes of opioid administration in the management of cancer pain, Oncology 1:10-18, April 1987.

Pilon RN and Baker AR: Chronic pain control by means of an epidural catheter, Cancer 37:903-905, 1976.

Poletti CE and others: Cancer pain relieved by long-term epidural morphine with permanent indwelling systems for self-administration, J Neurosurg 55:581-584, 1981.

Waldman SD: A simplified approach to the subcutaneous placement of epidural catheters for long-term administration of morphine, J Pain Sympt Manage 2:163-166, 1987.

Patient-Controlled Analgesia

Baumann TJ and others: Patient-controlled analgesia in the terminally-ill cancer patient, Drug Intell Clin Pharm 20:41-45, 1986.

Citron ML and others: Patient-controlled analgesia for severe cancer pain, Arch Intern Med 146:734-736, 1986.

Donovan BD: Patient attitudes to post-operative pain relief, Anaesth Intensive Care 11:125-129, 1983.

Fitzgerald P and others: Let your patient control his analgesia, Nursing 17:48-51, 1987.

Graves DA and others: Morphine requirements using patient-controlled analgesia: influence of diurnal variation and morbid obesity, Clin Pharm 2:49-53, 1983.

Kleiman R and others: PCA vs. regular IM injections for severe post-operative pain, AJN 87:1491, 1987.

Lukassko P: A guide to the parenteral management of moderate to severe pain, Hosp Pharm 22:361, 1987.

McCaffery M: Patient-controlled analgesia, Nursing 17:63-64, 1987.

Mioduszewski J and Zarbo AG: Ambulatory infusion pumps: a practical view at an alternative approach, Semin Oncol Nurs 3[2]:106-111, 1987.

Paice JA: New delivery systems in pain management, Nurs Clin North Am 10:715-727, 1987.

Rao MK and others: Evaluation of demand analgesia in a community hospital, Res Staff Phys 32:26-37, 1986.

Sheidler VR: Patient-controlled analgesia, Curr Concepts Nurs 1:13-16, 1987.

White PF: Post-operative pain management with patient-controlled analgesia, Semin Anesth 5:116-122, 1986.

Blood Administration

American Association of Blood Banks: Technical manual, Arlington, Va, 1985, The Association.

Bahu GAB: Administering blood safely, AORN J 37[6]:1073-1100, 1983.

Committee on Transfusion Practices, American Association of Blood Banks: The latest protocols for blood transfusion, Nursing 16[10]:34-41, 1986.

Grindon AJ and others: The hospital transfusion committee: guidelines for improving practice, JAMA 253[4]:540-543, 1985.

Kelting S and Johnson C: Erythropoiesis and neonatal blood transfusions, Matern Child Nurs J 12:172-177, 1987.

Landier WC and others: How to administer blood components to children, Matern Child Nurs J 12:178-184, 1987.

Pauley SY: Transfusion therapy for nurses: part 2, NITA 8:51-60, 1985.

Phillips A: Are blood transfusion really safe?, Nursing 6:63-64, 1987.

Pluth NM: A home care transfusion program, Oncol Nurs Forum 14[5]:43-46, 1987.

Rutman RC and Miller WV: Transfusion therapy: principles and procedures, Rockville, Md, 1985, Aspen Publishers, Inc.

Taylor BN and others: Development of a standard for time-effective patient assessment during blood transfusion, J Nurs Qual Assur 1[2]:66-71, 1987.

Chemotherapy

American Hospital Association Teleconference: Cytotoxic drugs; safe management through a team approach, Chicago, Oct 1986.

American Society of Hospital Pharmacist's Scientific Affairs Department: ASHP technical assistance bulletin on handling cytotoxic drugs in hospitals, Am J Hosp Pharm 42:131-137, 1985.

Barone RM and others: Intra-arterial chemotherapy using an implantable infusion pump and liver irradiation for the treatment of hepatic metastases, Cancer 50:850-862, 1982.

Barry LK and Booher RB: Promoting the responsible handling of antineoplastic agents in the community, Oncol Nurs Forum 12[5]:41-46, 1985.

Beverly S and Murphy B: Chemotherapy and home health care: special touch nursing, Kans Nurs 12:12-13, 1985.

DeVita VT Jr: Principles of chemotherapy. In DeVita VT Jr, Hellman S, and Rosenberg SA, editors: Cancer: principles and practice of oncology, ed 2, Philadelphia, 1985, JB Lippincott Co, pp 257-285.

Dorr RT and Ignoffo RJ: Extravasation of vesicant anticancer agents, Highlights on Antineoplastic Drugs 2:2-5, 1984.

Erickson K and DeBuque SM: Reaffirming catheter placement and patency, Oncol Nurs Forum 13[2]:14-15, 1986.

Eriksson JH and Swenson KK: Your guide to intraperitoneal chemotherapy, Oncol Nurs Forum 13[2]:77-81, 1986.

Garvey EC: Current and future nursing issues in the home administration of chemotherapy, Semin Oncol 3[2]:142-147, 1987.

Goldie JH and Coldman AJ: The genetic origin of drug resistance in neoplasms: implications for systemic therapy, Cancer Res 44:3643-3653, 1984.

Goodman MS: Cancer chemotherapy and care, Evansville, IN, 1986 Bristol-Myers Oncology Division.

Hood AF: Cutaneous side effects of cancer chemotherapy, Med Clin North Am 70:187-207, 1986.

Hughes CB: Giving cancer drugs IV: some guidelines, Am J Nurs 86:34-38, 1986.

Keller A: A CRNI's role in pediatric chemotherapy administration, NITA 9:466-468, 1986.

Lokich JJ and Moore C: Drug extravasation in cancer chemotherapy, Ann Intern Med 104:124, 1986.

Meadows AT and Silber J: Delayed consequences of therapy for childhood cancer, Cancer 35:271-285, 1985.

Meeske K and Ruccione KS: Cancer chemotherapy in children: nursing issues and approaches, Semin Oncol 3[2]:118-127, 1987.

Montrose PA: Extravasation management, Semin Oncol 3[2]:128-132, 1987.

Natale RB and others: Combination cyclophosphamide, adriamycin, and vincristine rapidly alternating with combination cisplatin and VP-16 in treatment of small cell lung cancer, Am J Med 79:303-308, 1985.

National Study Commission on Cytotoxic Exposure: Recommendations for handling cytotoxic agents, 1987, Providence, RI, Rhode Island Hosp.

Ommaya AK: Implantable devices for chronic access and drug delivery to the central nervous system, Cancer Drug Delivery 1:169-179, 1984.

Oncology Nursing Society: Cancer chemotherapy: guidelines and recommendations for nursing education and practice, Pittsburgh, 1984, The Society.

Pfeifle CE and others: Totally implantable system for peritoneal access, J Clin Oncol 2:1277-1280, 1984.

Tringali C: The needs of family members of cancer patients, Oncol Nurs Forum 13[2]:65-70, 1986.

U.S. Department of Labor, Office of Occupational Medicine: Occupational Safety and Health Administration: work practice guidelines for personnel dealing with cytotoxic (antineoplastic) drugs, Pub No 8-1.1, 1986.

Van Sloten HK and Aisner J: Treatment of chemotherapy extravasation: current status, Cancer Treat Rep 68:939, 1984.

Von Roemeling R and others: Chemotherapy via implanted infusion pump: new perspectives for delivery of long-term continuous treatment, Oncol Nurs Forum 13[2]:17-24, 1986.

Waskerwitz M: Special nursing care for children receiving chemotherapy, J Assoc Pediatr Oncol Nurses 13[2]:16-25, 1984.

Weinstein SM: Biohazards of working with antineoplastics, Home Health Care Nurse 5[1]:30-34, 1987.

Yarbro CH and Perry MC: The effect of cancer therapy on gonad function, Semin Oncol Nurs 1[3]:3-8, 1985.

Parenteral Nutrition

Aspen Board of Directors: Guidelines for the use of total parenteral nutrition in the hospitalized adult patient, J Parenter Enteral Nutr 10[5]:441-445, 1986.

Aspen Board of Directors: Guidelines for use of home total parenteral nutrition, J Parenter Enteral Nutr 11[4]:342-344, 1987.

Atkins JM and others: A nurse's guide to TPN, RN 49[6]:20-30, 1986.

Bender JH and others: Parenteral nutrition for the pediatric patient, Home Healthcare Nurse 3[9]:32-39, 1986.

Briggs BA: Nutritional support in the home, Oncol Nurs Forum 14[6]:79-80, 1987.

Cochran E and others: Principles of pediatric parenteral nutrition, Hosp Pharm 10:1014-1019, 1987.

Daly JM and others: Peripheral vein infusion of dextrose/amino acid solutions +20% fat emulsion, J Parenter Enteral Nutr 9[3]:296-299, 1985.

Dickerson RN: Question: how fast can I taper TPN in a hospitalized patient? Hosp Pharm 20[8]:620-621, 1985.

Ekman L and others: The glucose-lipid ratio in parenteral nutrition, Nutr Support Serv 5[9]:26-28, 1985.

Grimble GK: Administration of fat emulsions with nutritional mixtures from the three liter delivery system in TPN: efficacy and safety, Nutr Support Serv 7[10]:14-16, 1987.

Gulledge AD: Common psychiatric concerns in home parenteral nutrition, Cleve Clin Q 52:329-332, 1985.

Heymsfield SB and others: Anthropometric assessment of the adult hospitalized patient, J Parenter Enteral Nutr 11[5]:365-415, 1987.

Hogue EF: Management of legal risks associated with home health care, Nutr Support Serv 7[4]:23-25, 1987.

Irving M: ABC of nutrition, Br Med J 291:1404-1408, 1985.

Johndrow PD: Administer hyperalimentation in the home?, Home Healthcare Nurse 14:27-31, 1984.

Kovacevich DS and others: Association of parenteral nutrition catheter sepsis with urinary tract infections, J Parenter Enteral Nutr 10[6]:639-641, 1986.

Mauer EC and others: Lipid emulsion use in neonates and infants, Hosp Pharm 22:185-187, 1987.

Niemiec PW and others: Compatibility consideration in parenteral nutrient solutions, Am J Hosp Pharm 41[5]:893-910, 1984.

Ratliff M and others: Infection control in the home, Nutr Support Serv 1[1]:30-32, 1988.

Szwanek M and others: Trace elements and parenteral nutrition, Nutr Support Serv 7[8]:8-13, 1987.

Williams WW: Infection control during parenteral nutrition therapy, J. Parenter Enteral Nutr 9[6]:735-746, 1985.

Index

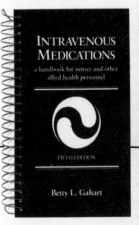